BEFORE PROTOCOL

BEFORE PROTOCOL

A FOOTBALL STORY

BROCK LUNDERVILLE

MILL CITY PRESS

Mill City Press, Inc.
2301 Lucien Way #415
Maitland, FL 32751
407.339.4217
www.millcitypress.net

Printed in the United States of America

ISBN-13: 978-1-54566-253-3

TABLE OF CONTENTS

INTRODUCTION

WHILE PLAYING FOOTBALL FOR MY HOMETOWN TEAM, I SUFFERED a tragic accident on September 15th, 1978. I was just a sixteen-year-old junior in high school—a defensive back for the Durand Panthers. In Durand, Wisconsin, like many rural areas in America, the community supports their local high school football. The small town, on the western side of the state, is snuggled between rolling hills and the banks of the Chippewa River.

In this book you learn of my story and although, at times, it may read as an almost unbelievable journey, these incredible events took place just as they are written. Many of the incidents probably should not have developed in the way that they did—some seem almost unfathomable. It is not my intention to embarrass or humiliate any of the doctors, nurses, or anyone else that helped take care of me. I consider myself one of the lucky ones… thankful that I am walking today. I could easily have been permanently paralyzed.

This story will take you on a trip through time, back to the fall of 1978 and early 1979.

This book is titled: *Before Protocol*, because it reveals the way sports were played back then. We played football... got hurt, and were rarely ever checked out or went to a doctor. If we were lucky, the team manager maybe taped your ankle or found some antiseptic spray to put on a cut. If you were playing high school sports back in the seventies, medical care or going to see a doctor was each player's responsibility. If you were hurt during a game, the expectation was that you should attempt to get back on the field and resume playing as soon as possible. It seemed there was more pressure to play while hurt, than it was to take care of the injury. That's just the way it was. Countless times, I witnessed my teammates continue to play with a severe injury. Back in the day when we had our *bell rung*—this is known today as a concussion—most often, you were expected to return to the game. Frequently, we inhaled smelling salts to stimulate the senses and ready the body for action. I can remember after one game, I was going to the bathroom. Another player walked by and said, "Hey... you're pissing blood?" I did not even realize it. A few days later, everything seemed fine. There were no nurses or trainers on the sidelines, we just had a manager.

I have no regrets about playing high school football; the accident happened and, at the time, I did the very best I could to deal with it. However, things could have and should have been handled differently. There was no training for coaches—there was no such thing as *concussion protocol*. Heck, the word *concussion* was rarely used. I also blame myself for not being sure of what was going on inside my body but still ignoring the warning signs. Fear of telling somebody that I could be hurt—not living up to expectations, and letting my team and family down, contributed to me keeping secret a few problems. Perhaps I should not have, but the warnings signs to me were just not clear. If I had to do it all over again, would I have played high school football? The answer is *yes*. I loved football and wanted to play. Sports were a large part of our family life and a part of our local community. Our small town was rich with sports history and I wanted to leave my mark. I wanted to follow in my brother's footsteps. This book will also give you an idea of what it was like growing up in a family of six while living in a small town.

Come along on my journey, as I reflect on one of the most worrisome and excruciating years of my life.

Chapter 1

GROWING UP IN DURAND

I WAS BORN 1961, IN DURAND, WISCONSIN—THE YOUNGEST OF SIX children. It has been said that last-born children tend to be the rebels, the daredevils, and the clowns… maybe because parents tend to relax the rules. I was definitely not a rebel or daredevil. However, I did have a little reputation as being the class clown in high school.

There were six of us growing up in a one-thousand square-foot home. My siblings were: Dixie, Scott, Jeff, Ross, and Tootie. By the time I turned eight, my oldest sister, Dixie, had left the nest and was married. Our home was situated just down the street from the high school. My mother, at age ninety, still lives in that house today. There were two small bedrooms upstairs and two more on the main level with one bathroom, a small kitchen, and the living room. There was no garage, not even an unattached one. With only one bathroom, there was usually chaos. No matter what, I was always the last one to bathe and, by then, the water heater had done its best, so the bath water was usually cold.

A family of six was actually a fairly common thing around the 1960s, especially in Durand. With the city's population around 2000, much of the sprawling countryside outside of Durand and along the Chippewa River was farm land. Families were generally larger, so there would be children to help with farm chores. The community also had a strong Christian faith.

Our house was always open; honestly, we never locked the doors, even when we went away. Back then, that was the norm. My parents never turned away a kid that needed a night's rest or a place to stay for a short time. It was not uncommon to wake up at our house and have people sleeping on the floor or laying on the sofa on the back porch. If my brothers were out partying and drinking and a friend was too drunk to drive, they just came to the Lunderville house.

In the early seventies, slow pitch softball was very popular and my brother Scott had a bar called *The 5th Quarter*. He sponsored a slow pitch team. I was the bat boy on the team, which allowed me to be able to be at every game and watch my brother Jeff play. I didn't want to miss a game and my brother knew it, so he always made sure I had a ride. If the team played late and some players needed a room, they had one at our place, again it was usually a spot on the floor or back porch on an old sofa, but they were welcomed. One time, my brothers brought home a guy—they told my parents he needed a place to stay for a while, that he just needed to get his feet underneath him and it would only be a short stay. The young man lived with us for about a year. It was no big deal—my parents were glad to help—even though it was another mouth to feed. I never heard my parents complain.

It is true that, being the youngest, the rules—for me—were relaxed. Growing up, even as a kid, I was on my own a lot. As a youngster, and with parents having full-time jobs, I seldom had a sitter. Even at the age of five and six-years-old, I was often left alone. That's what is referred to as a *latchkey kid* these days.

We lived in town and, during my childhood's sultry summers, I would ride my bike all over the place. It was orange with a banana seat with no extra gears, just the one. My dad got it for me from the local Holiday Store, complete with reflectors, as a birthday gift. The rule was, I always had to be back home by supper. I made plenty of stops at friends and the East Side Grocery , a small convenience store close to home. Frequently, I would buy baseball cards and enjoy the gum that came with the cards.

At a very young age, I enjoyed freedom. It seemed like everyone in town knew me and people were always friendly. On a typical summer day, as a youngster, I'd have little league baseball in the morning, either a game or a practice. Swimming lessons followed mid-day. In the afternoon, it was more sports—a group of my neighborhood friends would get together and either play baseball, football, or basketball. By the age of twelve, I had my first cortisone shot in my right arm—too much summer baseball. When we played sports, I always wanted to pretend I was my bother Jeff. We were ten years apart in age, so when I was seven, he was seventeen and a popular athlete in our town.

As a kid growing up, I worshipped the ground that my brother Jeff walked on. He was a high school basketball and football star and, more than anything, I wanted to be just like him. He played on championship football teams and his basketball team went to state in 1969 and 1970. At the age of eight, I was convinced that I was going to travel with my parents to see the State Basketball Championships at the Wisconsin Field House in Madison, Wisconsin. I would walk around the house yelling, "On to State!" "On to State!" I was so proud of him and his team for advancing to the state championships. A few days before the big games, my parents gave me the bad news: I would not be traveling with them to the tournament games, but would have to stay home. As a kid, I'd never missed a game. Left at home, I watched the state tournament games on a black and white Zenith television and ate Captain Crunch cereal. Seeing my brother on TV was exciting.

I can remember when my three older brothers got up for breakfast; my mom would buy the largest box of cornflakes cereal the store sold. My three brothers would eat the entire box amongst themselves. The same thing seemed to repeat itself at supper time. By the time the bowls of food got around the table to me, well… there wasn't much left. It was a constant chore for my mother to keep us supplied with food. It really didn't matter, because I was more interested in talking to my brothers about sports. I was always curious about football practices, and when the next game was, I did not want to miss it, especially watching Jeff play.

My mother was the planner, organizer and cook for our family. She worked outside the home and put supper on the table every night for six of us, after working an eight hour day. She helped us with school work in the evenings and made sure we had a lunch packed for school the next morning. She was continually flabbergasted that, no matter how much food she put on the table, it was always gone at the end of the meal.

At the young age of ten, Jeff and I found another bond. He bought me my first hound dog for hunting raccoons. I trained the dog by myself and began hunting with my brother—but then his college schedule interfered, so Jeff introduced me to Lynn Wittig, who became my hunting mentor. My Dad would drop me off at Lynn's place and we would hunt until 1:00 a.m. Even with the dark of the night, Lynn never used a compass; he used the stars, the moon and the lights from neighboring farms for navigation. I was continually amazed that we never got lost. Both of my coon hunting dogs were kenneled out at Lynn's home. My dog, *Boomer,* was a Blue Tick, and *Spider* was a Walker hound. Back then, you could make some pretty good money for raccoon hides, as they were turned into fur caps and coats. Lynn would skin the raccoon hides, dry them, and prepare them for market. One fall hunting season, between the two of us and our hunting dogs, we amassed fifty-three hides. That was our most profitable season ever. The hides were generally purchased by a Canadian Fur Trader. I have always loved sporting hunting dogs, training them, seeing them run on the hillsides, and wrestling with the raccoons. The money collected for the hides was just a bonus. My father's rule was: if I wanted to hunt until 1:00 a.m. in the morning, he was okay with it—as long as I got to school on time. No late night's hunting would be an excuse for missing school the next day or even being tardy. This was the Marine coming out in my Dad, the disciplinarian.

There was also plenty of commotion at our home, mostly the result of my brother Jeff's shenanigans. After two years, at two different division three colleges, playing football… Jeff dropped out. During his senior year of high school, he broke his ankle playing basketball at the state tournaments. This injury, combined with too much partying, cut his college career short. He also told me that he'd slacked off. His studying and class attendance couldn't compete with the partying. I once found a shoebox full of letters from colleges across the Midwest; they all wanted to recruit my brother. There were university coaches from North and South Dakota, Iowa, Colorado, and Wisconsin—all wanting him to play football. I was amazed when I read some of the letters and scholarships he was offered.

When he returned home from college, there was trouble. If a fight broke out downtown, at one of the local bars, it was like he could *smell* it. He was not afraid to take on more than one guy at a time. If the phone rang after midnight on a Friday, it was usually a call indicating Jeff had gotten into some sort of trouble. His knuckles were usually bloodied from fist fighting. His shirt would be in shreds and blood-stained. My dad would get so frustrated with Jeff's continual fighting.

At a young age, I became their mediator. I knew when Dad was pissed off and I would tell him that I'd take care of my brother when we got home from the police station. I'd clean him up… the blood and any wounds he had, and then soak Jeff's injured knuckles in vinegar.

"This bullshit has to end." My dad would threaten my brother, but the fighting never seemed to end. In reality, I think my Dad liked it that I tried to negotiate and stick up for my brother. I was only ten years old when my brother Jeff was twenty.

Shortly following one incident, I recall that I'd just gotten home from grade school, when there was a knock on the door. The county police stood there. Of course, they were looking for Jeff. He, along with my brother Ross, and some other buddies thought it would be fun to do a little fishing in the dark of night… in a closed trout hatchery pond. At the hatchery, during daytime hours, the public could observe the fish and even feed them. There was a gumball-type vending machine; you'd get a handful of pellets to feed the fish. The pond was never intended for public fishing, especially while they were closed.

Jeff's midnight fishing trip took place the night before our brother Ross was to leave to enter the Navy. This was a terrible night at the Lunderville home. After the intruders set off the alarms at the trout pond, the police arrived and surrounded the perimeter. Four young men were arrested and Jeff was nowhere to be found. He'd run for the hills. The cops released the bloodhounds to track him down. After about ten minutes of running in the dark, Jeff ran into a barbed-wire fence and split his head wide open. Rather than surrender, he continued to run in the dark—with blood oozing down his forehead and onto his chest. Despite the blood running down his face, and in his eyes, he recognized a friend's house. He knocked on the door. His friend's parents were woken in the middle of the night, but they took care of his self-inflicted wounds. They soon realized that he needed more medical attention than they could offer. They drove him to the local hospital, where he received at least thirty stitches across his forehead.

Sometimes my brother would actually be brought home by the local cops. They would just drop him off and not even charge him with anything. Weekend after weekend, especially in the summer, my brother Jeff could find trouble. He'd hot-rod around town in his car, speeding or just hunting for a fight. It was all part of the normal routine at our house. There was always calm after the storm at our place—despite problems, we were still a family. Given some time, life always worked its way back to normalcy. As the years passed by, I was ready to make the transition from grade school to high school.

Chapter 2

EARLY SEASON FOOTBALL

AS AUGUST OF 1978 APPROACHED, SO DID THE START OF FOOTBALL practice. Entering my junior year of high school, I was ready and determined to walk in my brother Jeff's athletic footsteps. The first few days were mainly conditioning drills, exercises, and running… fine tuning the players' bodies. We ran sprints, did pull ups, and slammed into tackling dummies. Some days, we'd have early morning practices, in anticipation of beating the extreme August afternoon heat. We usually had one or two guys become dehydrated or have heat stroke when the temperature climbed into the mid-nineties.

The first few weeks of practice seemed to go smoothly. We were getting slotted into positions and I landed a defensive back spot on the Varsity Squad—this was the spot I was hoping for. During my freshman and sophomore years, I played the defensive-back position, losing only one game out of both seasons. I loved to tackle, so defense was where I wanted to be. I enjoyed making contact and especially the impact from tackling. The team morale seemed high and Coach Pete Adler was doing his best to get us in shape.

In early August, we had a scrimmage against Menomonie at our home field. Menomonie High School was a much larger school, located about a half-hour west of Durand. We were holding our own against a much bigger school as we alternated series from the ten-yard line. This was a scrimmage format that was used for both teams to practice short-field defense.

Our opponent had the ball and they had moved to about the one-yard line. On the next play, they handed the ball to their fullback; he was a big kid. I met him head on. Like two rams colliding and locking horns, our helmets slammed against each other. The back of my helmet pinched against the back of my neck. Fellow teammates said they could hear the collision on the sideline. I nailed the guy and stopped him just short of the goal line.

My head ached from the forceful hit. There was immediate pressure on my head, and I felt a vibration travel down my left leg. I felt numb briefly. Then, everything moved in slow motion. I had no idea what was going on, but my head hurt. For some reason, there was a sharp pain tingling down my leg. My left arm had gone numb—almost like it was frozen. The numbing sensation would come and go.

Back in the huddle I used my right arm to cradle my left arm to ease the pain. I continued to play, but I was delirious. I can remember the other defensive back on our team, Ron Brenner, asking me questions and I had to grasp for answers. A few times he told me that I would just stare, unfocused and with a blank expression. He said I looked really dazed.

I didn't have much recollection after the goal line helmet-to-helmet hit. The rest of the day was fuzzy at best. I later asked Ron Brenner what happened on that play. He said, "You got your bell rung." Today, this is known as a concussion. I barely remember returning to the locker room to shower.

That same afternoon, my brother Scott was getting married. I was honored to be in his wedding. We had spent a lot of time together. I'd worked for him in his bar and learned a lot about running a business. I started working for him when I was in the fifth grade and continued throughout my college years. When I was younger, I cleaned bathrooms, emptied the bottle chute, mopped floors, and restocked coolers. When I was older, I bartended, cooked, and arranged booking live bands for the weekend, both Friday and Saturday nights.

After the head-on scrimmage collision, I went home and started putting on my tux for the wedding. I was struggling with my left arm; it did not want to cooperate. I was having trouble getting my shirt on. My arm was limp and lifeless. I had no idea why my body was so uncooperative.

"What is wrong with me?" Struggling with a basic skill, like putting on my shirt, left me puzzled, wondering why dressing had gotten so complicated. Not suspecting anything serious, I just kept quiet and asked my Dad if he could pull my shirt on and button the top button and help me with my tie. I told him I had hurt my left arm in the football scrimmage that morning and my arm was sore and had a pretty bad headache. He seemed a bit concerned that I could not lift my left arm very well, but he knew injuries came with football. It's a physical sport and I was a defensive back—it was my job to stop offensive players, sometimes by slamming into them or tackling the player.

During the wedding ceremony, my left arm started tingling. Then, intense and sharp pain ran from the back of my neck down to my toes. It felt like an electrical jolt. The sensation lasted for a minute, and then passed—but the headache lingered. It hurt badly. Again, in my mind, it was just a part of being hurt from playing football. Like in the past, I figured, *this too will pass*.

The remaining summer practices did not feel right. I was sore… but then, wasn't everyone? I thought maybe it was just my body, my muscles getting used to the heavy conditioning drills. My back hurt and the dull headache made its presence known constantly, it just never went away. I'd take a few aspirin and it seemed to help some, but the dull, aching pain continued. I remember feeling tingling in my fingertips and my arms, like small pinpricks. Not really sharp, just short prickling and tingling sensations. It felt like rain drops on my arms. One day, I talked to my mother about it, after I had ridden my bike down to see her at my brother's bar, where she was working. Trying to explain my problem, I told her it felt like it was raining out. However, since the sun was shining and there was no rain, she gave me an odd look and asked if everything was okay. So, I told her I was fine. But my arm and back were still bothering me from the hit in the scrimmage. In reality, I was getting a little scared, because the headache, the pinpricks and tingling… none of it made sense. But again, I tried not to make a big deal out of the nagging pain.

We opened our regular season in a non-conference game against Black River Falls. Our defense was good—we held our opponent to just six points, but we could not muster any offense, we were flat and did not seem prepared. The only points we scored were by our defense on a safety. Final score was 6-2, a loss. I felt okay in this game, but I was not able to completely *wrap up* on my tackles and my arms seemed a little weaker than normal. I still had the dull headache, but I was getting used to it.

A week of school followed and I was sluggish and began to experience nausea. I start eating less to ease the issue. It just seemed if I ate less, I felt slightly better.

Our varsity football team was preparing for our second non-conference game, this time against Arcadia. Our offense performed much better, putting up twenty-seven points and our defense again was solid, holding our opponent to just six points. I was hurting after this game. After a couple of tackles, that numbing pain ran down my back again, and it felt electrical when it surged down my leg.

After the game, I got on the bus with my helmet off, lingering there, in pain. Jody Brantner was a senior linebacker on our team; I called him *wild man*. He was as strong as they came—he would take down an opposing player any way he could, tackling a guy high, low, by the helmet or by ripping off their shoulder pads to bring the guy to the ground. Jody was vicious. As I sat on the bus after the game, Jody gave me a strong whack on shoulder pads, and said, "Hell of a game." I winced immediately and I could tell the pain revealed on my face scared him. Then, instantly, pain traveled down my left arm and leg.

"Are you okay, man?" he asked.

"Yeah, I'm okay." And I sorta was... a day later, when the pain seemed to dissipate and I went back to practice.

All of the other players on the bus hooted, hollered, and sang in celebration of our victory. I just sat by myself, my head leaning against the edge of the bus seat and the window. Shutting my eyes was the only thing that helped. I just needed quiet. The less I moved after the game, the less it hurt. Even though we had won the game, I had no joy. I had pain.

Opening up the conference schedule with a win was important; Ellsworth would be our foe. The game did not go as orchestrated. I could hear my brother Jeff hollering at me from the sideline, "Come on, Lunderville, hurt somebody. Let's see a hit." He continued to ride me. Then, midway through the first quarter, I had the perfect opportunity during a screen pass to their halfback. The opposing player caught the pass and was carrying the ball to his right side, leaving his mid-section wide open. I snuck around one lineman, and drilled the halfback right in his stomach with my helmet, completing the tackle and forcing a fumble. I could hear the wind as it was knocked out of him. The guy was hurt, there was blood coming out of his mouth. He lay motionless and eventually was taken off the field. He didn't return to play. I looked over at my brother and was wondering if he was happy, I'd just hit a player and hurt him at the same time. I was less than thrilled as the game was a replica of our first. Our defense played well, we put two points on the board with a safety, but our offense again could not put up points, we were defeated in our conference opener, 14-2. I had one deflected pass, a few tackles, and one forced fumble, but really made no impact plays. After the game, I ventured toward the opposing team as they were leaving the field—just to ask about the guy I'd hit. I was told that that he was better and the blood was coming from a gash on his tongue. I guess when I hit him; his teeth had pierced his tongue. I felt a little better about his situation, but still unsure of mine.

For me, the game was a killer. I had fatigue and may have been dehydrated. Maybe it was from not eating right. I felt like I was moving at half speed and couldn't figure it out. During the games, I wasn't getting to my opponents quickly enough and had trouble covering deep receivers. The numbing sensation was now down in my toes, a few times it felt like my feet were cold—they had a tingling sensation to them. The pain in my head had developed into a pounding headache and, every now and then, my eyes twitched. It wouldn't go away. I couldn't stop the sensation and had no idea what was causing it. My eyes would twitch at night while attempting to sleep. I'd lay there, staring at the ceiling, waiting for my eyelids to stop twitching, but it would last for hours. At that point, I was probably only getting about two to three hours of sleep a night. I figured a few days of rest would help, and then we'd prepare for our September fifteenth match up at home against Baldwin- Woodville.

If you could walk; you could play—that's the way it was.

Tomorrow is another day.

Chapter 3

THE HIT

SEPTEMBER 15, 1978. ALL DAY AT SCHOOL, ALL I COULD THINK OF was playing football. It's really hard to focus on school work on a game day, especially when you have a one-track mind, like me. Our team had a record of one win and two losses and we were opening conference play at home, in Durand.

The school day ended with a pep rally, and so our team was fired up and ready to play. We started preparing for the game about 4:30… guys getting their ankles taped or doing some stretching. A boom box bellowed music from Queen: *We Will Rock You.* After guys finished getting their ankles taped, they slid into their uniforms. As I put on my pads, Ron Brenner, one of my best friends and the other defensive back on our team, walked over and sat down.

He asked, "Who are we going to drop tonight?"

I replied, "Any of their receivers that we get a good run on."

Ron and I always got stoked up before a game. We'd played together on the playground as kids, and we both had gotten our tonsils out at the same time—when we were in the fifth grade.

Around 6:00 pm, the cool fall wind arrived, the temperature dropped, and the sun slowly faded. The lights went on at Wayne Field in Durand. *Friday Night Lights.* At six feet tall and 160 pounds, I played defensive back for our varsity team while still a junior in high school. Ron might have weighed 150 pounds wet. His nickname was "Goose Neck."

Before the game, in warm ups, I looked into the crowd and spotted my mom and grandma, they were both wrapped in blankets. I knew my dad had to work, but I looked over and noticed he was there, on the sidelines, wearing his work uniform. He was on the night shift and decided to take his lunch hour to watch the first quarter of the game. I knew he would not see the entire game, but just the idea that he wanted to see part of the game meant a lot to me. I was trying to see if I could spot my brother Jeff somewhere on the sidelines, but I didn't see him. I was a little pissed off that he might not be at the game. I'd really wanted him to be here. As a kid, I'd never missed a game he'd played in and damn it, I wanted him to watch me play.

The cheerleaders were busy, getting our crowd fired up for the opening conference game. One of the cheerleaders was Margaret Adler; her father was the head coach. After the game, she and I would be going on our first date. Yep, I was going to date the coach's daughter. I asked her to go out with me and she accepted. Nope, I was not sucking up to the coach; I had already earned my position well before I asked her out.

Our opponent that night was Baldwin-Woodville High School. As the game opened, we dominated, scoring early in the first quarter. I was having a good game, got a few tackles in and deflected one pass. Midway through the first quarter, my left thumb went numb—*completely numb*. I kept rubbing it in the huddles, but nothing… no feeling returned to my thumb.

I had great communication with Ron. We would always tip each other off about anything we observed. Halfway through the second quarter, I started to see the same formations and repeated plays. Our defense began to realize it, too. There was a short pass to the tight end and I had a good run at him. I'd tackled this receiver previously and he knew I could hit. The sweat dripped into my eyes and my vision started to blur slightly.

There was about ten yards between us. I had a straight bullseye shot at the opposing player's shoulder, but... somehow, I miscalculated. As I made the tackle, I lowered my head and the opposing player did the same. My helmet collided with the top of his—a direct collision—like two cars hitting head on.

My upper body completely arched backwards and my eyes looked up at the lights. It felt like my helmet had pierced through my skin. I hear a pop, a cracking sound, as I completed the tackle. Inside my head it was loud. I dropped to the ground and rolled over, then began to push myself up. My chin strap had become disconnected and my helmet was halfway off. When I got to my feet, immediate pain shot through my head. I felt tingling in my feet and fingers.

I wondered, "What is going on?" My vision was blurry as I worked my way over to the team. Staggering, I moved slowly and my teammates waved for me to hustle back to the huddle. They were ready to set our next defensive play.

Everything went bright white. My eyes rolled back in my head. Things seem to move in slow motion.

I could hear my teammates asking, "Are you okay?" and "Are you all right?"

"I can play... I think... I can play." Words came out of my mouth, but even I realized they sounded slurred.

Marty Weiss, our senior linebacker said, "Get him the hell out of here." Marty was as strong as they came. He grew up on a farm in rural Durand. He threw hay bales for summer training.

I was told to leave the field; but I was delirious...my vision was blurred. Everything seemed really foggy and I couldn't see straight. As I attempted to leave the field, I stumbled in the wrong direction, heading toward the opposing team. *Confusion... can't think.* I wasn't even sure what field I was on.

Our team had to take a timeout as we had too many players on the field. I had to jog completely across the field. Struggling to run, my legs were losing power. My left arm and leg would not keep up with the right side. I knew my coach was going to be pissed at me.

Coach Adler started coaching in Durand in 1961 and had a terrific winning record. At one time, our winning streak of thirty-six games in a row was the longest in the state's history.

As I neared the sideline, Coach Adler immediately confronted me.

He grabbed me by the face mask and shook my helmet back and forth yelling, "Lunderville, what is wrong with you?"

I must not have been able to answer quickly enough.

So, he hollered at me again. "What the hell is wrong with you?" He rattled my face mask a second time, looking for answers, I guess.

But I couldn't reply. I just stared... lost in a profoundly dazed state.

Finally, I managed to spit out some words. "Coach, it's my head...I heard a pop and a crack...got a headache."

Coach told me to go sit down on the bench. I tried to find the bench but was too weak. In a deep stupor, I couldn't seem to snap out of it. When the bench appeared in front of me, I collapsed onto it. Then, the pressure started building in my head, like an inner tube tire being over-inflated—but the air compressor just kept on pumping. The manager came over and cracked smelling salts then waved it in front of my nose. *Nothing*. I couldn't smell it.

I was numb.

John Hagness, our team manager, jammed the smelling salts up my nose further and drew blood. He said, "You don't look so good. Can you smell anything?"

I had no reply.

My feet were tingling and my arm was getting numb. *What is happening?* I couldn't think, couldn't figure it out. The pressure on my head was so strong. I began to heave on the ground in front of the bench. It felt as if there was an elephant standing on my head. It hurt to open my eyes. The intensity of the bright lights over the field were blinding, painful to me. I couldn't tolerate my eyes being open, so I squinted. It seemed like everything I looked at was bright white, or a silver color.

Our defensive back up for me, David Sinz—also a junior—was asking me all sorts of questions about our scheme and our defensive coverage. I attempted to tell him something but he didn't understand me. He just stared at me while I attempted to talk. My speech was so slurred I was incapable of communicating. Then, I felt a choking sensation in my throat. I just couldn't pull myself together. Double vision set in next and I got extremely dizzy. Things were still happening in slow motion and the noise, the crowd, the whistles, the cheerleaders... everything was way too loud. All I wanted to do was stay sitting down—it hurt too much to stand.

Shortly before halftime, we scored a touchdown. I heard the announcer say over the loudspeaker, "Touchdown, Durand!"

Mike hollered, "Showtime, Lundy." *Lundy* was my nickname in high school. Mike *Smitty* Smith was our field goal kicker and I'd always held the ball for him on extra points. He was a block of granite, about 190 pounds. He was a very close friend of mine. Mike and his dad ran a *Phillips 66* gas station in town, the kind where they still came out and pumped your gas.

My name was being called so I knew I had to get back on the field. Reaching for my helmet, I couldn't find it, so I took the nearest helmet and started to head onto the field. My left arm and leg were dragging a bit as I awkwardly approached the field. I knew I was late getting to the huddle, which meant another timeout. My coach was really upset now.

Pain shot from my neck all the way down to my feet. It felt like an electrical-vibrating sensation.

Still, Coach was furious.

"Coach, my neck… there is pain in my neck." I hoped like hell he wouldn't grab my face mask again. He told me to go wait on the bench and then head to the ambulance at halftime. Feeling nauseous, my stomach churned until I got the dry heaves again. That elephant was still standing on my head, it felt like my head might split open at any moment.

I walked over to the ambulance under my own power, even though I was dead tired and getting weaker by the minute. My footsteps were slow and unsure. I just wanted to sleep.

Nathan (Pit) Plumer was the ambulance driver. His son, Joe, was our quarterback and a very good friend of mine. Joe and I had grown up as neighbors, playing sand-lot baseball and football. There was already someone in the ambulance; a player from the opposing team laid on a stretcher in the back of the ambulance, he was being treated for a sprained ankle. He was there first so he got the stretcher. I was put in the front passenger seat with a neck injury. It didn't seem right, but I didn't care... I just wanted to go somewhere and lay down.

I looked out the front window of the ambulance before it pulled away from the stadium. I noticed a classmate, Joe Rhiel, watching me with concern. I wanted to talk to him, but I could not comprehend what was going on, still unable to pull myself together. He appeared blurry to me, nothing was in focus and I clenched my teeth in pain. As a precaution, they'd put a cervical collar on me.

I was taken to the local Chippewa Valley Hospital in Durand for examination. As the ambulance pulled away from the parking lot, the wounded player, from the opposing team, in the back on the stretcher began yelling about his ankle and the pain. I couldn't take his hollering. It hurt my head to listen to him. He continued to yell about his pain. I couldn't take his whining much longer, but he kept it up. My right shoe was loose, a Riddell football shoe, size ten, and I was able to get it off and into my right hand. I shifted to my left in the ambulance seat, took aim and threw the spike, landing it perfectly on his head. I shouted, "Shut the 'F' up." Finally, the inside of the ambulance was quiet—I just needed some silence. Just then then my stomach started churning, much worse this time. I was nauseous and having nothing to throw up in, I realized that God gave me two hands, so I used them to form a cup. I dumped the vomit out the window. My hands had stench from the vomit, but it was the least of my problems. The pressure on my head and neck were intense, my vision was blurry, and it was best if I shut my eyes for the remainder of the bumpy ride to the hospital.

Chapter 4

ARRIVAL AT THE LOCAL HOSPITAL

SEPTEMBER 15, 1978. UPON ARRIVAL AT THE HOSPITAL, I attempted to get out of the front seat of the ambulance but was struggling. Jason Schoonover, the other ambulance paramedic, assisted me out. My left arm and leg were still giving me trouble, they both dragged slightly. I was losing strength fast. In the emergency room, I was put on a flat stretcher. My neck had severe pain. The lights in the room were bright and I could barely open my eyes—the glare hurt my head even more. The pressure on my head was getting stronger.

The doctor entered the room and asked me where the pain was coming from. I pointed to my neck. They attempted to take off my jersey, but I winced in pain as I lay flat on my back. I asked for a pillow or cushion to put under the back of my neck. The medical team decided it was best to cut off my jersey with scissors. To me it seemed like simple steps were taking forever. The next issue was my shoulder pads. As they attempted to pull them off, a sharp pain ran down my back and I clenched my teeth in pain and I actually let out a scream. The pads were finally unlaced and slid off to the side of my body.

The X-ray Technician was Ellen Adler, she was the coach's wife and I was supposed to be dating her daughter tonight. Sort of like *All in the Family*. Yes, this was small town America.

Several X-rays were taken of my neck and head area. My eyes were heavy and I dozed off while lying on the flat, hard X-ray table. No idea how long I slept.

I heard a voice and it was the Doctor, David Castleberg.

He said to me, "Brock, the best we can tell is that you have a sprained neck, it is sometimes called Whiplash."

I was glad to hear that was all that was wrong with me… there was nothing broken, so that made me feel comfortable. I would be kept in the hospital a few days, for observation. I was still very nauseous with a severe headache. The tingling in my feet and hands hadn't gone away either. As the nurse rolled me onto a gurney, the sound of the wheels and the rattling of the cart were killing my head.

Every little noise was like a firecracker going off in my head. *I guess this is what comes with a sprained neck, hopefully it will go away*.

I was assigned to a room. My body smelled like a locker room. I was told I would not be able to take a shower immediately, as it was more important to lay flat and rest. My arms had grass stains and my hair was soaked with sweat from my helmet. I still wore a jock strap, a pair of gym shorts, and the short sleeved T-shirt I had on under my shoulder pads.

Tylenol was administered for the pain. Even after my *nap*, I was still drowsy and felt my eyes wanting to roll back in my head. An uncontrollable twitch began on my whole left side. I couldn't move my head to the left—there was strong, immediate pain if I tried. My head wouldn't completely turn to the left without locking up. This, again, I assumed came with a sprained neck. I went back to sleep but was interrupted. It was my mom; she seemed more worried than me at this point. Her eyes were filled with tears. She told me she had spoken to the doctors and was aware I had a neck injury of some sort.

She'd brought a bag with clean clothes for me. Her worried expression gave away her concern for my condition.

Lord, what is happening here? Things are not normal, I thought to myself. I have never felt this way or felt this much pain. Right after my mom left, my date for that evening, Margaret Adler, came in, I was slightly embarrassed—I smelled, felt, and looked like shit. *Not very impressive for a first d*ate. How embarrassing. She was also aware, after checking with her mother—who'd taken the X-rays—that I had a neck injury.

I began to apologize to her... we would not be going on our first date. No downtown Durand to Bud's T-Birds, where young people gathered after the game for a cheeseburger, French fries, and a cherry Coke.

Bud Sperger, the owner, made the best burger in town. On Friday nights after a football game, he probably made 200 burgers and fries. You could shoot pool and play foosball with friends. There was a juke box—three songs for a quarter. It was just a good place to hang out and stay out of trouble. That was the Friday night ritual after every football and basketball game.

I remember Margaret looking at me and I knew she could tell I was hurting; my eyes were still watery from talking with my mother.

"Well I messed up our first date."

She assured me that we would do a makeup date at some point, it was more important that I rest and get better. I could barely hold my eyes open… I just needed to sleep, but I asked her one last question. "Did we win the game?" She looked at me with a grin and said, "Yes, we won the game." I managed to smile back. I told her that I had asked for a radio to listen to the rest of the game on our local WRDN channel, but the nurse did not think it would be a good idea. The doctor wanted my room to be quiet and calm. I began to doze off and I don't remember Margaret leaving the room.

Later that night, I could hear a rumble through the window in my room. It was a familiar noise—a sound I swore I'd heard several times before. Although it sounded like thunder, it reminded me of a car engine revving up for a drag race. The sound started coming closer and louder, it seemed like it was coming from the parking lot. I was groggy and confused about what I was actually hearing. I attempted to open my eyes, but I could feel them roll back in my head. There was a very large wall clock in my room located near my bed, but I could barely see it, the time appeared to be 1:00 a.m. in the morning, but I wasn't sure. What would possibly be going on outside the hospital at that time of the night?

Suddenly, I heard the door to my room open, but I couldn't see very well, since my room was completely dark. I could hear somebody stumbling around and talking to a nurse. Then my room filled with fumes, it smelled like a Kentucky Whisky factory. The smell became stronger and seemed to be right on top of me. I opened my eyes to the sight of my brother, Jeff. His face hovered directly over me and the smell of alcohol woke me. He had driven his 1974 Dodge Charger right up to the front door of the hospital and revved up the engine to get the attention of the nurses on duty. He wanted to be let into the hospital to see his kid brother. The entry doors were locked—it was well past visitation hours. Regardless, someone let him in so he wouldn't wake everyone in the facility. I guess someone downtown, at one of the watering holes, told him that I had been taken by ambulance to the hospital so he thought he would pay me a visit after the bar closed. I could tell he had been drinking heavily, Corby's and Coke was his drink of choice and he could put a few down. My brother informed me that it was important that I get better, and it was imperative that I play in next week's game. He tried to be positive, repeating over and over, "You can come out of this," and "You can play."

He was getting choked up and his eyes teared up. I asked him if he was at the game, I wanted to know if he had been at the game. I would be pissed if he wasn't, so I kept pressing him for an answer. "Were you at the game?"

He stuttered and stumbled for words and finally told me that he got hung up downtown at the bar a little too long. I stopped talking to him. He could tell I was hurt, deeply hurt. Not only were my feelings hurt that he was at a bar instead of the game, but I was hurt physically. Having my brother there to watch me play would make me proud, but tonight that feeling was hollow because he wasn't there. He reached out to shake my hand but I couldn't lift my arms, I was too weak and sort of numb. Jeff looked confused and concerned that I couldn't shake his hand, so he reached down and lifted my hand up and gave it a shake. I winced in pain. He told me later that it was then that he realized I was really hurt and in pain. After a ten-minute visit, the nurse came in my room and said that my brother needed to leave, as she could get in trouble for letting him in the hospital at that time of the morning. I was worried that he was going to get in his car and drive again after drinking, but he always seemed to make it home no matter what. Jeff agreed to leave and, as he pulled away, I noticed blood on his hands. I could faintly see his battered knuckles. He was trying to hide them from me. I just assumed he had been fighting again downtown, nothing out of the norm for a Friday night.

After letting my brother out of my room and relocking the hospital entrance doors, the nurse returned to my bedside and noticed blood on my bed sheets and wanted to know if I was bleeding.

"No, I am not bleeding." I told her it probably came from my brother's battered hands. The bloodied sheets were left on till morning. I began to drift back to sleep, but my headache lingered and I started to vomit again. Each time I heaved, the wrenching movement brought pain to my neck and head. It was an incredibly long night—it just seemed like it would never end. That day, up until then, had been the longest of my life. I just felt sleepy and so weak. I hoped that tomorrow would be a better day.

Chapter 5

A CRY FOR HELP

SATURDAY, SEPTEMBER 16, 1978, AT THE DURAND HOSPITAL. I woke up in the morning and was in a different room. Somewhat startled and a little confused, I had no recollection of being moved to a different room in the night. I must have been in a deep sleep when they transferred me. There was still soreness in my neck and I couldn't move without aching, but the vomiting had eased. I felt like I had been through a war. I still couldn't move my head to the left, my neck would literally lock up, and it just would not turn. *This doesn't seem right.*

Even though I couldn't turn my head, I noticed I had a roommate. He was told by the nurses of my neck injury in last night's football game. The guy's name was Gerald Hunter, a big guy from Durand. His nickname was "Beef." With a name like that, you can well imagine that he was a big guy. I think he weighed around 300 pounds and had big, broad shoulders. His forehead was pronounced, along with his chin, but his eyes were sunk back in his head. He was a member of the county police force. He told me he was having chest pains and they were going to look him over. He did not seem extremely worried; he felt they were taking precautionary measures. It seemed to me he was breathing very heavy and I could hear a gurgling sound in his voice when he spoke.

There were visitors in and out of my room most of the day… family, friends, and teammates. They offered encouragement all day long that I was going to recover and things would be okay. The assurance that I was going to be okay was encouraging, but I was really starting to wonder, "Am I *going* to be okay?" The day was long, too.

Later in the afternoon, the hospital posted a "No Visitation" sign on my room. Our room was to be quiet and I needed some silence, but *Beef* began telling me stories of all the great football players Durand had in the 1960s and 70s. I was listening, but so very tired. His stories seemed endless. He asked me questions about last night's game and my injury but I was not very responsive. I informed him that I had a helmet-to-helmet collision and hurt my neck and that the doctor told me it is a sprain.

Drowsiness overcame me. My eyes start to flutter and I slowly drifted off to sleep again. I started to dream. I had no idea how long I slept. My dream was filled with trouble... someone was struggling to breathe, the person needed help. I could hear a man gasping for air. I needed to leave this troubling dream—it was too realistic. I somehow woke up and realized I was not dreaming. My roommate, Beef, was having trouble breathing. I could hear a buzzer going off. The only thing I could do was attempt to roll—like a log—in my bed so I could see him, since my head wouldn't turn to the left. Once I got rolled over, I could see there was trouble.

There was a loud pop, like the sound of a pin popping a balloon, and a gigantic gasp for air. Was he having a heart attack? How long had I been asleep? How long had he been gasping for air? His chest looked swollen and he was shaking. He was choking and turning blue. It looked like he had hit his buzzer for a nurse. *Where is a nurse? This man needs help fast.* I tried to hit my buzzer—my damn fingertips were still numb, I couldn't get hold of the buzzer. I finally pulled my right arm over to the edge of the bed and hit my button for a nurse, and hollered as loud as I could, "Help!" I was in pain from lifting my neck to scream, and was about to yell again, but finally, the nurse arrived and I pointed to Mr. Hunter. He was not looking good. His hands twitched and he was still gasping for air.

Deep heavy gasps, as his body rose up and down off the bed. He was turning blue in front of me. The gasping went shallow and then he looked lifeless.

There was mass commotion in the room. They announced a *code blue* and a doctor and other nurses ran into the room, all working on Beef. He was eventually taken to the emergency area.

Left alone now, I was nervous, then broke out in a full-body sweat. Then, I felt water running down my face. My bed was soaking wet. I was worried and a bit rattled. I was hopeful that they can save the man's life, but it looked grim. I have never witnessed anything like that in my life.

My room was finally silent, but I could still hear commotion from the hallway. Eventually, a nurse came by and shut the door to my room, which left only dead silence in my room. I started to wonder what was happening outside my room. *Were they able to save my roommate?* It seemed like hours went by. Due to nervous tension, sleep evaded me… I need to know what happened; my concern for him was all-consuming.

After a while, the doctor walked in my room. "How are you feeling?"

My reply was that I was not feeling good. I had a sore neck, headache, and tingling in my toes and fingers. The doctor took an instrument and scratched the bottom of both of my feet. Toes on both my feet wiggled and he indicated that was a good sign that I still had feeling. The doctor then pricked a few fingers, and I had feeling in both hands.

At that moment I really did not care about myself, I was more concerned about my roommate. "What happened to Mr. Hunter?"

The doctor looked at me and said, "We lost him. He is no longer with us."

I just stared at the doctor. "He's dead?"

"There was nothing more you could have done, Brock. It was a massive heart attack. Our team did everything we could to revive him."

I was speechless; I do not know what to say. A guy that was telling me stories thirty minutes before was gone. The doctor informed me that he will send in a nurse to clean me up and give me some medicine to help me rest. A man I'd just barely met for one day died in my room. I will never forget that day as long as I live.

I was hoping things would get better; surely, they cannot get any worse. I felt terrible about the situation and was overcome with guilt and pain. I started wondering, *how long had Mr. Hunter been gasping for air? What if I hadn't fallen into a deep sleep and heard him sooner? What if I could have hit my emergency buzzer sooner?* Over and over I kept searching for answers, but came up empty.

Chapter 6

FAILING

I WAS SERIOUSLY FAILING LYING IN THE HOSPITAL. I WAS STILL shaken up about Beef's death the day before and it was hard to put it behind me. There was now something going on in my throat—like a knife, jabbing me every time I swallowed. In response to the irritation in my throat, I stopped eating to avoid the pain, I could barely swallow water. I thought I was bleeding in my throat, but no blood, just pain.

Sunday night I got electric-type tingling up and down my back, I couldn't sleep, thrashed my feet in bed all night. The day was long and the night was even longer. I was worried that something was seriously wrong; I had never felt this way before. In my mind, there was no progress—only failure.

On Monday September 18th, the nurse suggested that I get up and take a shower. The doctor had given me approval to get out of bed. I was in favor of this as I had not been able to bathe since being admitted. I smelt like a pig and my hair looked like I had greased it back with Vaseline. Even though it hurt to walk and there was pain in my neck and left leg, I wanted to get cleaned up. A good hot shower might make me feel better. I could only take small steps, due to the pain in my back, but I made it to the shower. While I was in the shower, I noticed the shower head could be removed and had a massage setting. I took the showerhead and massaged my neck for about fifteen minutes, pulsating water over the back of my neck. It felt good. The more I did it; the better it felt. Back and forth I went with the massaging shower head. The hot water seemed to ease some of the pain. I was using my right arm to wash my body. Drying off was a complete struggle but I finally managed. As I stepped out of the shower, I noticed a large mirror. As I glanced in the mirror, I could see that I did not have good color—I was pale and peaked. I was also given a toothbrush and, as I opened my mouth, I noticed my tongue was all white around the outsides, I did not ever remember my tongue looking like this before. Brushing my teeth felt good… but something else was happening. My tongue had started to get *thick* on me, like I was losing feeling in it. I managed to crawl back into my hospital bed, but things were definitely not right. By late afternoon Monday, I noticed that I was having a little difficulty speaking; my tongue just did not want to cooperate. A friend and teammate, Pat Baier, stopped after football practice with a malt from our local Dairy Queen. I was happy to see both him and the ice cream. I took a spoonful of the malt and started choking, startling Pat. He gave me a very concerned look and eventually left to get home in time for farm chores. I then told both the doctors and nurses about the situation, and they noticed my speech was slower and not as clear. My throat was also starting to go numb and I was choking on Jell-O and even water. I was really concerned. *Does all this stuff really happen with a sprained neck?*

I woke up on Tuesday September 19th. It had now been four full days since the neck injury happened and I was having difficulty speaking with the doctor. My words were not coming out the way they should. He had a puzzled look on his face. I wasn't getting better; everything seemed to be getting worse. I asked the doctor if they could call my mother and let me speak to her and he agreed. My mother answered the phone and she was having trouble understanding me, too. At first, she was confused who was on the phone.

"Mom, I need help." But she didn't understand me as my words came out sounding mumbled. My tongue was thick and getting in the way. I asked my mother to please get Dad up to the hospital; I really wanted to get to a different hospital. She could tell I was having difficulty speaking; my words were slow and slurred. She said she would call my dad at work and see if he could come up and get me. My tongue was stiff and turning white upon my dad's arrival.

The doctor agreed that there was something they were missing; they should transfer me to Eau Claire- Sacred Heart Hospital for further medical evaluation. This was a much larger hospital with newer and more sophisticated X-ray equipment. It was about a thirty-minute drive from Durand.

When we went to the front office to sign out, my father was informed that there were no ambulances available, they were both out on emergency calls. No ambulance… that almost seems impossible. The only thing my dad could do was check me out and drive me to Eau Claire in his own car. I was walking slowly out of the hospital, carrying a small pail, in case I needed to vomit. The nausea was back again and there was severe pressure back in my head. Under my own power to the parking lot, feeling faint, and dragging my left side, I fell by the side of the car, landing on the pavement. I couldn't get up on my own. My body was just too weak. I kneeled, holding on to the car door. My dad picked me up in his arms. My head and neck dangled as he laid me flat in the back seat of the car with my puke pail. That was a good idea—because the vomiting started again.

Chapter 7

HOSPITAL TRANSFER

TUESDAY, SEPTEMBER 19, 1978. MY DAD WAS GIVEN INSTRUCtions to first take me to an X-ray clinic, located adjacent to Sacred Heart Hospital in Eau Claire, about a half-hour's hour drive. X-rays were taken while a tube was inserted down my throat. I was having a lot of pain opening and closing my mouth while they worked at getting the proper X-rays.

"Just one more X-ray, Brock." They tried to reassure me, but the procedure seemed to never end.

My eyes watered from the pain. *What are they looking for if I only have a sprained neck?*

After several hours of X-rays, we were instructed to go back to the hospital. All the way back to Durand we went, another thirty-minute car ride and more sickness. My head pounded and my vision began to blur. Then the vomiting started again.

Upon arrival back in Durand, nurses met us at the front door and instructed us to immediately head *back* to Eau Claire Sacred Heart. "Go to the emergency room entrance," they stressed.

This is crazy, I thought to myself. Somehow, there was a miscommunication. I have now had X-rays for three hours and been in the car for over an hour. And we're not finished. As I walked to the car, I fell again, overcome by extreme fatigue.

My dad helped me up and put me in the back seat. Here goes my third car ride of the day. I was lying flat in the back seat and I could tell that my dad was tense and having his patience tested. Apparently, the X-ray clinic in Eau Claire thought we had already checked into the Sacred Heart Hospital next door, we had not. So, when they instructed my father to go back to the *hospital*, all the way back to Durand we went. While my dad drove, he stewed over their communication failure. When he got mad, he also became very quiet. Twenty minutes into the venture back to Sacred Heart hospital, we were nearly back to Eau Claire, when I heard my Dad yell, "We got a blow out in a front tire." I heard gravel hitting the car, knew we were heading for the ditch and my Dad hit the brakes. Our car skidded—then I felt us veering off the road. I rolled off the back seat and fell onto the rear floor as the car jerked to a sudden stop. There was instant pain as I was pinned in the floor of the car. The vomit from the pail covered me and my shirt plus the car seat. The smell was terrible… gag-inducing. I struggled to work my way back up on to the rear seat, but couldn't see my father. Just then I heard him holler from outside the car that he needed me to help change the flat tire. I honored his request, however, I moved in very slow motion.

Our car had stopped—but was about to go over an edge into a ditch. My Dad had jacked up the car, but he also had to push against the car so it does not tip further and slide over the edge. He instructed me to lift the tire and push it onto the axle. I could barely stand. I felt shaky, then wavered and almost fell into the ditch. Finally, I managed to push the tire on and my father tightened all the lug nuts, throwing the bad tire and wrench, with vengeance, back into the vehicle. By the sound alone, I could tell my father was pissed off. I told my Dad that my body was going numb, losing more feeling.

"We are only ten minutes from the hospital, hang in there, sonny boy. We will be on Highway 37 real soon," he said.

Arriving at the ER, nurses and doctors were waiting for us. Struggling to walk, I reached for my Dad for help. The medical staff was amazed that I was not sent in an ambulance. I overheard one nurse say, "Look, he is walking on his own." Two other nurses and one doctor immediately strapped me down to a gurney. Sand bags were put all the way around my head.

Sandbags?

My dad seemed a bit confused. I had no clue what was happening or why. Another doctor walked over and introduced himself.

"Mr. Lunderville, I am Dr. Mike Ebersold. I have to give you some bad news… I have read all the X-rays. Your son has a broken neck."

A broken neck? What? People die from that, I thought. My father walked away, I lost sight of him. Where had my dad disappeared to? Over a minute went by, and my dad got a grip on his emotions. He paused and eventually returned and looked over me.

A tear fell on my face.

I had honestly, never once, seen my dad cry—not once. For the first time ever, I saw a worried look in his eyes. Even when his own mother passed, he was as strong as a rock, he never cried.

I looked up at him and the only thing I could think of to say was what I'd heard the past few days. So, I repeated it, "I am going to be okay."

The doctor informed us that surgery would be performed sometime soon. I was admitted to Sacred Heart hospital in Eau Claire on September 19th, 1978. A broken neck at level C1-C2, meaning my first and second vertebrae was broken. It was far more serious than a sprained neck.

I asked one of the nurses if people can die from this and she said, "Some people do, but we are going to take good care of you, Brock."

Chapter 8

DELIVERING BAD NEWS

SEPTEMBER 19, 1978. DAD DECIDED THAT HE WANTED TO DRIVE back to Durand and give my mom the bad news face to face; my father never liked the telephone. If he had bad news, he wanted to say it in person to my mother—that is just how my father dealt with things. I knew she was not going to take it well.

My father left me alone but, before leaving, gave me a gentle pat on the leg. "The doctor is going to fix you up. They are working on some sort of plan."

Then I was moved in a special elevator that would accommodate the stretcher. Flat on my back with more sandbags on my head, I was immobilized—completely strapped down to a flatbed gurney. Even my arms were held down tightly. I thought about my car rides back and forth between cities, bouncing around in the back seat...

falling to the floor, lifting a tire. That kind of activity was the total opposite of how they were treating me now.

I was assigned to a male nurse. He pushed me on the flat cart and I could hear a lady crying in the background. She was going to ride on the same elevator. Then her crying got louder and louder. The noise was hurting my head. She was sobbing and having trouble holding her composure. I finally decided to ask her, speaking while staring straight up at the ceiling. “Ma’am, why are you crying?”

She leaned over me, looked directly down at me and said, “My son was in a cycle accident, he broke his neck and they called me to tell me he died. I am going up to see his body.”

I was left speechless. She wanted to know what was wrong with me; I told her that I just found out that I’d broken my neck playing football. She reached for my hand under one of the straps and held it the rest of the elevator trip. It left me unsure if I was giving her comfort or she was comforting me. Either way, it was some comfort.

We exited the elevator and I was left in a hallway, underneath a very bright light, still lying flat on my back and unable to move my neck or arms. The bright light made my head hurt, so much pressure on my head. I begin to sweat heavily after what I'd just heard, wondering if I was going to die. The lady just told me that her son died from a broken neck, so maybe I was next in line. I listened to as many things as I could hear in the background. There is a lot of movement in the hallway and I could sense some chaos. The only thing I could see was the ceiling and lights, but I could hear. Close by a nurse's station, I heard two of the nurses say, "We lost another patient. Room 218." I could barely look down the hall with my eyes turned as far as I could turn them. I could faintly see a white sheet, draped over a body on a bed. The lady that rode the elevator with me was crying over the body... her son was dead. Even a glimpse told me her face was wet—drenched with tears.

A few days earlier, a man had died in my room. Now another person was dead. They wheeled the bed and body past me in the hallway. The lady paused and looked directly down on me. Her tears landed on my face. She gave me a kiss on my face and whispered in my ear, "May God Bless you." I never knew the lady or got her name, but she cared. When she spoke to me, she was very sincere and genuine. I choked up, not knowing what to say in response. I laid there on the stretcher, totally speechless.

The nurse came to move me. My room was ready...room 218-2. The thought hit me like a bolt of lightning. That was the room where people died. Now I really begin to worry. Another person was dead. This was so far from my normal existence. Anxiety, tension, and fear ran amuck through my mind.

Chapter 9
DECISION

SEPTEMBER 20-21, 1978. MY DOCTOR WAS CONSULTING WITH DR. Onofrio at the Mayo Clinic in Rochester, Minnesota. It's the top medical facility in the Midwest. My X-rays were sent there for observation and a second opinion. It had been six long days that I have actually laid with a broken neck. The doctors were speaking cautiously as I was told that a break at the C1 and C2 level are extremely touchy and the surgery is delicate. My mind interpreted: *dangerous*. I was informed that the doctors were looking at two options to repair the break: flatbed traction or halo traction.

The nurses wheeled me up to an area of the hospital and showed me a patient that was fixed to a flat bed. You are basically immobilized and bolted to a flat board. You become a patient at the hospital for three months, under complete nursing care the entire time. To me, it looked like some form of punishment. I could not imagine not getting up to go to the bathroom or being able to leave the bed. One of the nurses also told me that body sores were an issue from being left in one position for such a long time. The patients I was able to view looked miserable. It scared the crap out of me. It did not look like anything I wanted to be involved with. Choosing this option meant missing school for three months and repeating my junior year of high school. I had already missed a week of school and certainly did not want to miss three months.

Ninety days in the hospital was not for me. I was taken to physical therapy where I could observe a couple patients with halo traction. These patients were upright and able to walk. A halo traction cast was basically a body vest—mine would be lined with sheepskin wool for interior padding. The vest would be connected to metal bars and a halo ring around your head, held in by four pins that are drilled into your skull. It looks like your body is in a cage. The pins are visible and you can see them piercing into the skull. As bad as halo traction looked, it was better than option one. Being able to at least walk and return to school and not fall behind was important to me. This option made the most sense and both doctors and my parents came to an agreement... halo traction it would be.

As I was being wheeled back to my room, I could see my brother Ross down the hallway. He was with Dr. Ebersold and they entered my room together. I was immensely happy to see my brother. He was working at a hospital in Rice Lake, Wisconsin, about an hour north of Eau Claire. He was a surgical technician at the time. I had no warning of this unexpected visit, but it was great seeing my brother, it was one of the few times I was able to smile. He was the one in our family that had medical knowledge and the fact that he cared brought tears to my eyes.

The doctor confirmed again that he'd looked over the X-rays one more time and that traction was best way to heal the broken vertebrae at C1 and C2 level.

It was then that my brother explained to me just how severe my injury really was. He was able to view the X-rays with the doctors. When it comes from someone in your family, it really hits home. I could tell that he had been in conversation with the doctor about the severity of the injury and the treatment plan. Surgery would be scheduled for September 23, 1978, a few more days to wait in pain.

Chapter 10

A VISIT FROM A STRANGER

SEPTEMBER 22, 1978. BY NOW, THE WORD HAS SPREAD BACK home that I would be having surgery, so I had a lot of visitors—family, and friends—the day before it was scheduled. It seemed news traveled fast in our small town. There were people in and out of my room all day during visitation hours. The doctor suggested that my room be off limits the night before the surgery and wanted me to get plenty of rest, so, at 7:00 p.m., my room was posted "No Visitation." I was beginning to doze off… and then something very strange happened about 8:00 pm. A minister walked into my room. He appeared to be a priest, since he wore black clothes and the white collar. His hair was long on the sides and curly on top and some shade of grey. He approached my bedside and wanted to know what happened to me. I told him I broke my neck playing football. The man had a slight Irish accent. The priest started telling me football is not a good sport, and he started ranting and raving and putting down football. He told me that Rugby was a better sport… on and on he went.

If I could have raised my arms, I might have punched him. I thought to myself, *Who sent this guy here and why did he stop to check on me? I don't even know him.*

Then something very bizarre happened. He held his left arm up high and looked straight up at the ceiling. He uttered some sort of Gregorian chant. *We never sang like that in my church.* I was a little worried at this point. *Who is this man in my room?* He never gave me his name or anything. What was going on here? His chant softened and it's like he was having a conversation with God in the form of a song. Startled, I was about ready to push my button for a nurse, because this shit was scaring me. Then his right hand was held straight out, pointing directly over me as I lay in bed.

Then he said, "If this young man shall die, lift him up to you, Lord." He made the sign of the cross over me and told me good night. My eyes were about to bulge out of my head… now I was scared shitless. I had no idea what to think. The man walked away after the blessing and shut the door to my room behind him. I was still trying to get my head around what has just occurred. I took my right hand and reached down inside my underwear; checking to make sure I hadn't messed myself.

About a half hour later, the nurses came in and reminded me that surgery will be performed very early in the morning. They began to take vitals and draw blood. My arms had marks all over the place and they were running out of veins to tap into. I started a conversation with the nurse.

"Did you see the priest that just left my room?" I told the nurse that he gave me some sort of a blessing as he sang to me. She laughed at me. "What did he sing?" I could tell she was in disbelief, but I told her it was some sort of Godly chant. She said they had kept a close eye on my room and nobody had entered as far as the nurses station could tell. I knew there was a priest at the hospital, so I just assumed it was someone from Sacred Heart. They told me that the chapel priest was actually gone for few days. No clue, no idea, not a dream, just a very strange event. I was so scared... *could I actually die? How serious is this? Who sent this man to my room?*

Chapter 11
SURGERY

SEPTEMBER 23, 1978. ABOUT 6:00 A.M., I SLOWLY WOKE UP. THE diagnosis on the medical report read: fractures at lateral mass of C1 and C2 and the spine was not in alignment.

It had been seven days since the injury occurred. Dr. Ebersold appeared and informed me that he would begin surgery very soon. I was alone in my room until a nurse came in to give me 100mg of Demerol through the IV to make me sleepy, but not totally knock me out. I was shocked when the nurses told me that the surgery would be performed in my room. Immediately after the IV kicked in, I got drowsy… very tired.

I was hoping they would wait. I really wanted to talk with my mom and dad, but they decided to move the surgery to an earlier time, so I would not be able to see my folks 'till later that day. I drifted off into a deep sleep, feeling like a balloon floating in thin air… blissfully, there was no more pain. I was up in the sky, floating on a soft white cloud, but could faintly hear nurses murmuring in the background. My eyes were too heavy to open. I was totally pain free and in a new, welcomed comfort zone. Even though I was completely asleep, I was able to sense a smell in my room. Not sure at first what it was, but then it hit me. It reminded me of the time that I'd scorched my hair over a campfire when I was in the Boy Scouts. Burnt hair… the terrible smell got stronger. I was semi-conscious but still unable to open my eyes.

Then, a witch came into my room, with very long fingernails, and poked me around my eyes. First the left eye, then the right eye. In my mind, I wondered why someone was poking me with their fingernails. There was more poking and scratching. I heard some sort of motor—but couldn't make a connection. I was startled and decided it was time to leave the cloud. I struggled to open my eyes, but there was something coating them.

Finally, I opened my eyes and discovered two doctors, who were leaning over my head holding a drill; my skull filings were coming out of the drill bit and landing on my eye lids. That smell was not burnt hair, it was burnt skin.

This was no dream—it was real.

I felt heavy tension and pressure being put on my head, the elephant was back and he was sitting on my head. Extreme pressure... the doctors were using a torque wrench to insert the pins into my skull. I shut my eyes and gladly went back to my dream. When I awoke, I was in a cage. Four holes had been drilled into my skull, two in front and two in the back sides of my head. Screws were inserted and attached to the halo traction body vest. This contraption was to immobilize my head and neck and align the vertebrae for healing. For three months I would be in this cage. I felt trapped inside my body, inside the cage.

Chapter 12

PHYSICAL THERAPY

SEPTEMBER 24, 1978. THERE WAS A NEW PATIENT, NOLAN, assigned to share my room. He was to undergo physical therapy also. My guess was he's about 30 years old. My understanding from the nurse was that he'd fallen thirty feet, from atop a ladder while working construction. He landed directly on his face and shoulder, shattering bones in both places. The accident had robbed him of his hearing also.

Initially it was thought that Nolan had broken his neck like me, but he was lucky from that standpoint. I had to learn how to function with the Halo traction and so began physical therapy. I had been lying in bed too long. They told me that it was time to get up and get moving. Two nurses assisted me out of bed for the very first time. When I got to my feet, dizziness overwhelmed me. The unfamiliar weight of the halo almost tipped me over as I was pulled forward, but the nurses grabbed me before I fell.

The weight was so heavy that I felt the nausea building. I couldn't hold it back and I covered one of the nurses in my vomit. It was an embarrassing situation. I felt like an idiot. My vision was blurry and my body was suddenly top heavy. The second nurse had a good grip on me and started walking close by my side. I had no idea how heavy the halo was, I wobbled, but got a bit steadier with each step. After a walk up and down the entire hall, it was time for physical therapy. I had to learn how to roll like a log for getting in and out of bed, then, how to bend over without falling down. I was shown different ways to get in and out of a bath tub and had to practice this repeatedly. After three sessions of intense physical therapy all in one day, my body was depleted. The nursing staff seemed to think I was on the right track and looking good in physical therapy. I was told that I may be able to go home in a day or two. I was ready to get out of the hospital; just the thought of hearing the word *home* made me feel better. Back to family and friends and my own bed.

The whole ordeal had left me weak and exhausted. I had very little appetite and found it very hard to swallow wearing the halo. Because of the position your neck is placed in, the esophageal muscles were not fully functional. I found that out in a hurry. I was choking on all my food, even drinking water was difficult. My mom's home cooking was sounding better and better. But I now knew that eating and swallowing would take patience and learning.

Dr. Ebersold checked on my progress and was extremely pleased with the physical therapy reports. He wanted to meet with me and my parent's tomorrow afternoon. I prayed to the Lord that I would get out of the hospital. Still, the days were long and the nights were longer.

Chapter 13

THE LUCKY ONE

SEPTEMBER 25, 1978. IT WAS EARLY IN THE MORNING AND I heard some sort of scratching on the door of my hospital room. At first, I thought it was a nurse or cleaning lady. Somebody was struggling to get the door open to my room. I was lying flat on my back looking straight up at the ceiling… about the only thing you can do with a halo on. The door finally opened, but I could only see the top of the person's head, and it looked like a midget. I had my eyes turned as far as I could, trying to look over the empty bed next to me when I heard a voice. "Brock, it's me… David."

In my mind, I was trying to place this voice. *I know this voice, I have heard it before. Can you come closer please?*

"Look at me Brock, it's me, David." I used the motion they just taught me in physical therapy and I pushed my head up on two pillows so I could see who was in my room. It was David Bauer, a guy from my high school. He had been in a bad accident in the early summer of 1978, after graduation. There was a party at Lake Eau Galle, near my home. David and his friends had floated picnic tables out in the water. They began diving off the tables, but unsure of the depth of the water, David ended up diving into shallow water, hitting his head on the hard bottom of the lake and, as a result, he broke his neck. He had severed his spinal cord. I was somewhat startled as David came closer to my bedside. I could clearly see that he was in a wheelchair. He asked me how I was doing. I told him that I may be going home soon. He asked me to wiggle my feet, so I did. He told me that he would never be able to use his feet or legs again... he was paralyzed, never to walk again. The injury had crippled him.

He wished he could take one night back in his life. He wished he could do it all over again, just erase that one night. He began to tear up. I was lost for words, so silence filled the room.

All I could tell him was that I was sorry. I remember going to school with him and I knew his family. Why and how can two young men from the same small high school both break their necks? David had to leave the room as he was having some medical testing done. He started for the door and then spun back around in his wheel chair and said, "You are the lucky one."

I must admit I got pretty choked up and a few tears slowly rolled down my face. *God, I am lucky*, I thought to myself. It really could be worse even though I thought it could not. Maybe being in halo traction for three months was not so bad. At least I could walk. *I was really lucky, David was right.*

The only other person I knew that was paralyzed and in a wheelchair for life was my Grandmother. Shortly after that my doctor appeared. "Brock, it's time for you to go home. I have called your parents and they are on their way to get you.

The journey home.

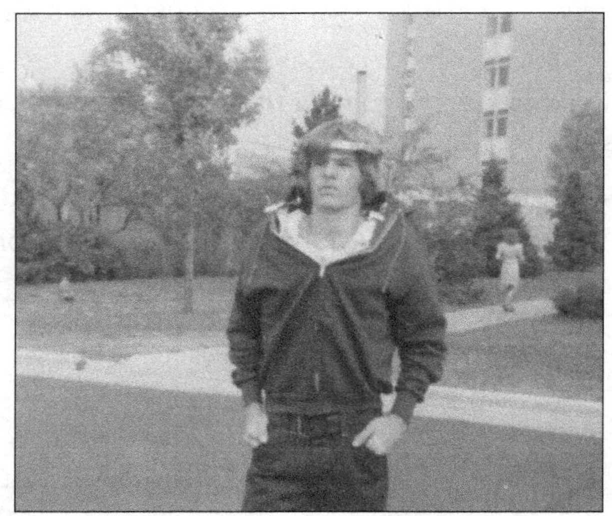

Brock leaving the hospital in halo traction.

Chapter 14

RETURN TO SCHOOL IN HALO TRACTION

SEPTEMBER 27, 1978. I WANTED TO GET BACK TO SCHOOL AS SOON as possible and was sure I was ready to return after missing a few weeks. Our home was located on East Washington Street, right across from the high school, so I was able to walk to school every day and build up my strength. When I arrived at school, I got many strange looks, most of the students had never seen anyone in halo traction and it kind of scared them. Margaret Adler seemed concerned that someone could run into me or knock me over in the hallway, but I assured her I would be fine. I went to the office in the Durand High School and gave the school secretary my medical excuse. She was writing me out a pass to return to classes, when in walked the assistant principal. No *Welcome back.* Instead he said, "You have missed a lot of school and my understanding is you have makeup work." I acknowledged that both statements were correct and that I would get all my homework caught up and that I had already started some of it. Under my breath I was really thinking, *What a jerk.*

I was not looking for a hero's welcome or anything like that, but not to even ask how I was doing or feeling. *For crying out loud, I broke my neck playing at a school athletic event.* I went about my business and returned to class. It all seemed fine for two to three hours and then I hit *the wall.* I became very weak and peaked. I had to return to the main office and inform them that I needed to go home; I did not have the energy to continue the day. Here came the assistant principal again, asking me all sorts of questions. I told him that I would give it my best tomorrow to complete a full day. After getting a pass to leave the building, I noticed the door was open to the gym. I needed to sit and rest anyway, as I was about to collapse. I had stopped at my locker and picked up my basketball shoes, just the idea of carrying my shoes made me feel better. I was bound and determined I would play sports again. If there was a will there was a way. I wanted to be on the basketball court by winter.

I could hear the bell ring, bringing the next class in session and then there was total silence. While everyone else was in class, I sat on a bleacher in the gymnasium all by myself. I just needed to rest for a few minutes. I stared out at the basketball floor and wondered if I would ever play again. I couldn't imagine school without sports. I shut my eyes and dreamed of making a long shot from the very far corner. I could even hear the crowd roar as the shot went in. "Basket by Lunderville," from the announcer. I had practiced the shot the entire summer of 1978, it was a shot I had seen Todd Doverspike perfect in 1973, today it is known as a three-pointer. If there would have been a three-point line back then, Todd may have held a state record. My brother Ross was a teammate of his. I could visualize coming down the court, drifting off to the far corner and having Joe Plumer or Ron Brenner hit me with a pass and pumping a rainbow jumper. After sitting for ten minutes, I wiped a few tears from my cheeks and began my walk home with my homework by my side. The halo cast was heavy and I was still very weak, overcome with fatigue. All of my school teachers were very supportive and helpful with my makeup work and tests. Tomorrow was another day... I hoped it will get better.

Chapter 15
SEVENTEEN

OCTOBER 26, 1978, I HAD BEEN IN TRACTION FOR THIRTY DAYS; but it had seemed like a year. My seventeenth birthday was today, in my halo, or as I called it, "my cage." Never in my wildest dreams did I ever think I would be in this condition on my birthday. I was only getting a couple hours sleep a night, the halo created problems for me in bed, and there is nothing comfortable about it. Applesauce, pudding, and liquids were the core part of my diet. At one point, I even ate some baby food because it was easy to swallow. The halo cast was lined with sheepskin so I was always hot. Not to mention, I constantly itched. I found that a fly swatter worked well to reach up inside my body vest and scratch like crazy. Every day I had to extend the metal handle of the flyswatter under the body vest and scratch with it. Sometimes I noticed blood oozing down to my waist line. My mom and my sister Tootie became my full-time nurses. My sister's real name was Eileen, but nobody ever called her by that. I guess when she was born my older brother had trouble pronouncing her real name so he called her "Toot-Toot." She then inherited the name *Tootie* and, in essence, it became her name.

The screws going into my skull had to be swabbed twice a day with Betadine. I was not allowed to shower, only a bath from the waist down and dab a wash rag on my arms and face. My sister washed my hair with dry shampoo; no water could touch my head. We were warned not to get an infection in the area where the pins were drilled in to my skull. I never knew there was a product called dry shampoo, it was in a spray bottle. My sister sprayed it on, then let it dry and combed it out. My daily wardrobe was a pair of jeans and an XL hooded sweat shirt, the only thing we could find to fit over the body vest. Homework was about caught up and I seemed to be back on track, except for eating, which continued to be a problem—an issue that haunted me. Because I only got a few hours' sleep at night, I'd doze off now and then in class.

Terry Thornton, a friend of mine, gave me a little nudge now and then to keep me awake, and if slept too long, he'd give me his notes from the class. There were always classmates that had my back.

All my pants were falling off my waist since I was losing weight. I struggled every day with swallowing. My little nieces and nephews were afraid of me—my halo frightened them—so they kept their distance. They thought I looked like Frankenstein. Everywhere I went, people stared at me in my cage, but I got used to it. I mark off each day on a calendar, waiting for *halo removal day*.

My doctor told me sometime in December, they would take a look at my neck and take more X-rays to confirm alignment and healing.

As for football, I made it back on the sidelines to spectate the last couple games of the season. Just being with my teammates made me happy. Basketball practice was close to starting and I continued to carry my shoes with me, in hopes of being back on the court in December or January. I never gave up hope!

I was getting encouragement every day from my classmates: Joe Plumer, Ron Brenner, Mike Smith, Kyle Bauer, Don Myers, Pete Komro, Ivy Schlosser, Luanne Talford, Diane Fedie, Jeff Moore, Joe Rhiel, and many more. Each day somebody gave me a boost, just when I needed it. The days were long and the nights were still longer. *But someone has it worse than me,* I would tell myself. *Move forward and do not feel sorry for yourself, tomorrow will be brighter. Something good had to come of this, right?*

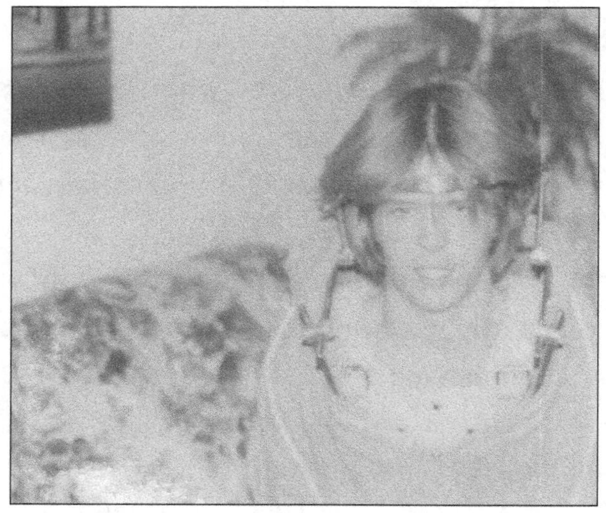

One month into wearing halo traction.

Chapter 16

RAINING ON A SUNNY DAY

NOVEMBER 1ST, 1978. OCTOBER PASSED AND NOVEMBER FOLlowed, with old man winter approaching. The temperatures fell below freezing and my walks to school were cold, but I did not mind. The morning breeze that flowed through my halo vest seemed to cool me off and get rid of some of the smell that had accumulated inside the body vest. The pain seemed just to be a normal part of my day. I tried to make the best of it. My lower back was getting sore—my guess was the weight from the halo cast caused it, or maybe the inability to stretch my back.

After supper one evening, I decided to listen to some music. I sat at the kitchen table and had just finished doing some school work. I had put in one of my favorite 8-track tapes, Creedence Clearwater Revival (CCR), I was listening to John Fogerty sing, "Have you ever seen the rain, coming down on a sunny day."

Reflecting back on a typical day in the summer of 1978—there was football practice, working for my father painting houses, and working at the 5th Quarter Bar, the business my brother owned in Durand. I rode my bike a lot and almost every day went to see my mom at work.

From August until the time school began, I'd started telling my mom that I could feel rain drops on my arms, just a light mist. One day I'd told her I was sure it was raining out.

She walked outside with me to verify and told me, "The sun is out, there is no rain."

Unsure of what I was really feeling I just kept quiet and to myself. I thought, *It didn't hurt, so why complain?* It seemed like every day after football practice there was that tingling feeling on my arms, but it was only ever on my arms. I also noticed that I had this feeling more when I rode my ten-speed bike and bent over and then looked up with my neck, that was when it rained the most. Why and what is this feeling? I wasn't really sure, but I was sure that it could rain on a sunny day.

Chapter 17
THE FALL

NOVEMBER 18, 1978. I WAS HOME ALONE AND WAS ATTEMPTING to take some steps that led from our house entryway to our back porch. For some unknown reason, I lost my balance. I guess I was a bit dizzy. Unfortunately, I missed a step, fell forward and crashed into a wall *with my halo on*. I then fell backwards heading down our basement stairs. My left leg was bent sideways; it felt like I'd torn something in my leg. The top rear of my halo was caught on the very top step; the only thing that kept me from falling down about twenty steps to a cement floor was my left leg which was pinned under me and my halo. If I fell down the steps and into the basement, I was going to be a mess… or die.

Holy shit, this is bad. I know that screaming for help wasn't an option—no one was home. Lying flat on my back, I looked up and noticed some jackets hanging in the hallway above me. My immediate plan was to slowly lift my right arm up and grab one of the jackets. As I started to grab the coat, the snaps unbuttoned, *damn it*. Maybe this plan was not going to work. If the coat came off the hanger, I wouldn't be able to get up. My path would be straight down to our cellar floor.

I began to sweat as I knew this fall could be deadly. If I slid down the steps or went over the edge of the stairs, the party would be over for me. In my head, I prayed that I could keep pulling myself up. I was running out of power, but I knew I had to get up. I gave one more tug on the coat. The very last button stayed snapped on the coat and I was able to get myself upright.

I was rattled and decided to just sit there for several minutes to pull myself back together. I immediately noticed two things. My left leg was starting to swell around my knee where it had bent sideways. I could feel the swelling tightening inside my blue jeans. The knee began pounding, bringing with it intense pain. The second thing I noticed was that the front pins in my forehead had popped loose from the halo .I knew this was not good. I could feel the pins moving in and out of my head. I was sure that I needed medical help, but not sure yet what to do.

I hobbled on one leg to get to the phone, trying to balance my body on one foot in a halo cast was no easy feat. I was able to contact my sister-in-law, who drove me to Sacred Heart Hospital in Eau Claire.

My doctor was making rounds and he met me in the emergency room. He asked me what had happened. I just told him I lost my balance and my halo bumped a wall. I kept it simple but not entirely honest.

He told my sister-in-law and me that he would re-attach the pins with a torque wrench and to prepare for pain. As he reached for the wrench, a nurse gave me small block of wood to hold and she told me to clench it if I needed too. The first turn of the wrench brought immediate pain and tears from my eyes. The pressure was so strong I felt faint.

The doc said, "Three more turns, Brock, and we will have the first pin in, then the second pin."

Water poured out of both eyes, there was nothing to numb the pain. The block of wood dropped from my hands as the pressure eased, it was over, the ratcheting sound had ceased. My fingers had left several gouge marks in the wood. The good news was the doctor did not see any damage, and he told me that I should come back on December 8th.

"Brock, it is time for us to take a closer look at your neck and take the halo off at your next visit. If all goes well, you will be out of your halo for Christmas. Then, your next step will be a cervical collar." Although there was terrible pain all the way home, it didn't matter. I did not care. My sister in-law was attempting to carry on a conversation with me, but I stayed quiet... really quiet. That was a close call; it could have been the end if I would have fallen fifteen feet down into the cellar.

December 8th was all I cared about. "Free to get out of my cage."

Chapter 18

THE SNOWMOBILE RIDE

FRIDAY, DECEMBER 1, 1978. I HAD A TERRIBLE DAY OF SCHOOL. My face was flushed with heavy sweating most of the day, I had no clue what was causing it. I had walked the short distance home and began sweating even heavier in cold winter weather. There was sweat running off the front pins in my skull and down the side of my face. The perspiration was dripping down inside my halo vest and the sheepskin lining was beginning to itch. Inside the medicine cabinet, I found a thermometer. My temperature read 103. Holy crap, I knew this was not good. I had to somehow find a way to cool off. I put ice in a washrag and rubbed it all over my face, but it did not seem to be helping. By then, my forehead was actually very hot to touch. I was burning up with a fever... maybe I had an infection. Just when I had run out of ideas, I glanced out the window and noticed that it was snowing. The ground was already completely covered and the roads had snow on them also. I spotted our two snowmobiles out in our back yard. I was getting anxious to take a ride once my cast was off. It was then that it hit me; maybe I should see if I could get one of the snowmobiles started and ride it up and down the street and let the winter wind cool me down. I was only one week away from getting my halo off and was not sure if this would be a good idea, but it was an option. *The decision was made.*

I found an old pair of boots on our porch and put another jacket over my halo. No idea if I could get one of the snowmobiles started, but it was worth a try. I thought I would give the 1974 Chaparral 440 a shot, it was my sled. The machine needed to be pull-started, so this was going to be a challenge. I put the choke on and pulled two times, but the engine would not turn over. As I sat on the seat and rested, I thought I would give it just one more try. I took a deep breath, and with both hands, I pulled the rope. *Rumble, putt putt, rumble…* what do you know? The damn thing had started. Three times's a charm.

After letting the machine warm up, I took the sled slowly up and down the street two or three times and opened up my jacket and let cool air flow into my halo vest. The cold wind whipping across my face brought gratification. My long hair was flying back and forth and I caught snowflakes with my tongue. I could feel my temp going down and I was no longer sweating… mission accomplished.

As I rode past a few of my neighbors, they look at me perplexed and confused that I was out riding on a snowmobile with a body cast on. The longer I rode the better it felt. After a twenty-minute ride, I put the snowmobile back in place in our yard. It seems the ride was the answer. As I was putting the cover back on the machine, I noticed my mother had arrived home from work. She was wondering what I was doing out by the snowmobiles. I told her that I noticed one of the covers had blown off and went out to put it back on. I did not dare tell her that I went for a ride. I knew if my dad found out, he would be pissed about the situation, so I never said a word. I said a prayer that night that none of my neighbors would tell my mom or my dad about the ride. It must have worked, because I never got in trouble.

Chapter 19

REVERSE

FRIDAY, DECEMBER 8TH, 6:00 A.M. I WAS UP AND READY TO HEAD to the hospital in Eau Claire. Today was the day I get out of my cage—the halo body cast was coming off.

"Get in the car, son, and let's get this damn thing off you. I am getting sick of seeing you in it," said my dad. All I could think of on the car ride was what it will feel like to move my head and neck again. It would be nice to get back into normal shirts and clothes. Not having to lay in a halo cast and be sore and immobile every day. *What would it be like to get a normal night's sleep?* I really wanted out of the body cast for Christmas.

My dad, being a man of few words, just said that he was hopeful that I would be able to play sports again someday and I agreed with him. I knew football was out of the question, the doctors had already told me that. Upon our arrival at the hospital, the medical team removed the pins from my head with the wrench, they certainly felt better coming out than they had going in. Next, they unstrapped the body vest, but put sandbags around my head to prevent any movement. I was wheeled on a flatbed down to radiology, where over twenty X-rays were taken. After that, I was then sent to a waiting room, still lying on a flat bed. All I could look at was bright lights glaring down on me.

An hour went by and my dad was getting nervous. “Why aren’t they telling us anything?”

I started to sweat and get tense. I knew growing up as kid, good news came fast. This felt like eternity; I swear we were there half a day waiting. “What’s taking so long?”

Finally, after a very long wait, Dr. Ebersold appeared from the far side of the waiting room. He came close to my flat bed and said, “Mr. Lunderville and Brock, I have some very bad news. Your neck is still broken, it did not heal. There is bad alignment at the C1 and C2 level and we are now worried there is abnormal pressure being put on the 3rd and 4th vertebrae.”

I had no idea what to say or do. I just looked up at my dad—he shook his head and said to the doctor, “What now?”

I had no clue what this news meant. I never considered that *not healing* could ever be an option.

Doctors needed to do surgery immediately. It was time critical to get the spine aligned and get the upper neck healed. The doctor had contacted Dr. Kennedy to assist in the surgery. He was anticipating operating in a few hours. "This is not any easy operation as we will be dealing with the spinal cord," he said.

My Dad couldn't believe what he was hearing and I just laid there, speechless.

"We need to get Brock admitted to the hospital and start running tests immediately. Mr. Lunderville, please stop at the front desk and sign the papers allowing me to perform emergency surgery. Brock, I will be back to see you in about an hour."

My dad looked down at me, just staring. "I will go back and get Mom and hopefully we will see you right after surgery." He reached for my hand and said, "Hang in there." It was one of his most common things he told us when things got tough, *just hang in there*. As Dad left, I was being transferred to a different room, still lying flat on the bed. Water began to flow down from my eyes to the sides of my face. I wondered if I would be alive for

Christmas. I started to think about being in a wheelchair and what I would do if I was paralyzed; so many things started rolling through my mind.

A nurse came in and took blood and all my vitals. All the same stuff over and over again. The door to my room opened and I could tell it was a new doctor.

"I am Doctor Kennedy. I 'm going to work with Dr. Ebersold today and we are going to put you back together. We're going to go into your strongest hip and cut out a few pieces of small bone, these bone grafts will then be inserted in the fractures and between your first and second vertebrae. After that, we will then insert wire and wrap them around both the vertebrae and create a fusion."

Both doctors looked at me and asked me if I had any questions.

"What about my hip, will I be normal? Will I still be able to walk?"

"You're going to have a nice-sized scar on your right hip, but you will never know we took bone grafts from the area."

As they told me this, I wondered if they covered all of this with my dad. I had never heard of a fusion, so it was all new to me. The doctor left the room and another nurse came in with a big black marker and started making marks on the skin of my right hip.

"This is where the doctors will take the bone from, your right hip as your right leg is your strongest, according to the tests we did," she efficiently explained.

Minutes later, the door to my room opened and in walked my classmate Jim Britton. He was in the hospital getting X-rays on his nose and getting checked for a concussion. Jim had taken several flagrant elbows to the face in basketball and had broken his nose several times. It got so bad that he had to wear a hockey goalie mask while playing basketball. Jim walked over to my bed and asked me how things were going. I gave him the bad news. I told him that my neck hadn't healed. My voice cracked with nervousness. I explained to Jim that when they moved my neck during the X- ray process, they found the fractures were still there. Jim couldn't believe it. He had a confused look on his face and, really, who wouldn't have?

He put his hand on my left shoulder and stared down at me. There was a minute there, where you could have heard a pin drop… dead silence. We talked for a while and he told me that he would go back to school and tell everyone to pray for me. He and my dad were the only two people I'd seen that day before they put me under. I just remember how we both got choked up and could barely talk.

Some time passed and I was alone again. The phone in my room rang, I could barely reach the cord on the phone, but I managed to get the phone to my ear. All I can hear is someone crying loudly but no voice, it got louder and then a pause, "This is your mother, I am so sorry for you. We will see you after surgery and are praying for you." As I hung up the phone, I stared at the ceiling, wondering what was happening. This was not going according to plan and things were moving way too fast.

Just then, a priest appeared in my room. I had never seen this priest before. I honestly do not know or remember his name, but he was very nice. He told me that he wanted to bless me before surgery and asked for my permission. I asked him to bless me, because I needed all the help I could get, especially from God. The Father said a very long prayer and then he stood by my bed and made the sign of the cross. He told me that anytime an emergency surgery was performed and he was in the chapel, he would always try to visit that person and bless them.

It had been about an hour and the phone rang again. This time, it was my grandmother and I could tell she was shaken up, even more than me. She was crying and telling me that she loved me and hoped that everything turned out okay. My grandma was at the game the night of the injury. She's always cared about me. As I hung up the phone, the anesthesia doctor appeared and informed me that it was time to start giving me some medications through an intravenous drip and that will start making me sleepy.

Just after that, my neurologist, Dr. Ebersold, entered my room and told it to me like this: "Brock, it has been a long haul for you and, unfortunately, your neck did not heal properly. But we are going to put you back together again. You will have limited range of motion after this surgery, but I am hopeful you will have a normal life." Both doctors were looking over me with the operating room team.

Breathe deep and count to ten, the lights in the room are so bright, "One, two, three, four…"

"How are you doing Brock, how are you doing?"

All I could hear was *beep, beep, beep.*

Chapter 20

RECOVERY

SATURDAY, DECEMBER 9, 1978. "BROCK WAKE UP... PLEASE, CAN you wake up?" I felt someone tapping me on the face. I finally woke up; as I looked up, I could see my doctors. They told me that they wanted to have a long talk with me. It was 8:00 a.m. in the morning and I was alone again. I do not remember anything about the afternoon of the surgery and then, I had slept through the night. There is some sort of new cervical collar around the back of my neck and up around the front of my chin. Dr. Ebersold first told me that I would be in the hospital for close to a week.

He added, "We can take no chances this time, we have to be completely sure your neck is going to heal and that we have good alignment."

I was worried about missing more school, but I did not say anything to the doctors. Dr. Kennedy wanted to know when my parents would be back to the hospital. He wanted to discuss the surgery. I told both doctors that I did not know when my parents would be back, but I thought maybe later in the day. They both looked at me and said that they felt it was important to tell me about the surgery.

"Brock, we noticed some very... *unusual*... things when we operated. We found two small fractures in your neck that were already starting to heal on their own. They did not show up on the X- rays." They also noticed a crack in the back of my skull and were surprised that this had, also, started to heal.

I couldn't believe what they were telling me.

"We have operated on several patients and have never come across anything like this. Brock, we need to ask you something... can you ever remember having a concussion or major neck pain before this last accident?"

I was silent for a while, and then I decided to spill my guts. I went on to tell them that I remember hitting a guy helmet-to-helmet, back in early August in a scrimmage against Menomonie in Durand. After the hit, I had tingling in my hands and feet and I had a severe headache and I did not remember the rest of the scrimmage.

"Can you tell us more?" they asked.

"I remember playing in some games and making a tackle and having pain run down my back and there was a light vibration for a few days, it seemed like my headaches were constant. I played in four games with non-stop pain, and then the final hit, it was like no other."

"Brock, we are convinced you broke your neck prior to this accident. What happened was, your neck was weak and trying to heal from the previous break and your spine could not sustain the last blow, but it fractured in a different spot."

Dr. Kennedy looked at me and said, "You had someone looking over you, I have never seen anything like this before." Both doctors told me that they would check me daily and, once the sutures in my neck and hip started to heal, they would remove them, and make sure no infection was evident. I would then be allowed to go home in a "Philadelphia Collar."

"We need to get you moving immediately to avoid blood clots—we want to start you walking today."

The doctors left the room, so I decided to go to the bathroom. I walked pretty wobbly, having gotten so used to being top heavy; my body had to re-learn balance. Without the halo, I felt much lighter. I had the urge to scratch up under my gown; there was irritation from the previous Halo cast. I turned on the light in the bathroom and spotted a large mirror and could not believe what I was seeing. My skin was so pale. My hair was long and greasy. I was as white as a ghost. There was a bathroom scale under the sink and mirror, and I decide I would step on it, but it was very difficult for me to look down and see my weight with the new neck collar on. I arched my back and the scale said I weighed 142 lbs. *Can this be right? Have I lost eighteen pounds?* I decided to reach back and untie my hospital gown, the ones that have no back and your butt cheeks are exposed. As the gown dropped down, I again looked in the mirror, there were three pinkish stripes going across my chest. Not understanding what these marks were, I edged closer to the mirror and realized that my ribs were showing through my skin. I resembled the likes of a skeleton. I remember taking the fly swatter and scratching up inside my body cast and must have worn off several layers of skin. There were four large, body sores on my chest, oozing with puss and blood. I had no idea what my back looked like.

I called for a nurse. I'd seen enough for one morning. The nurses applied salve and dressed the infected areas. When my mom and dad arrived that afternoon, I told them that everything was fine and I was hoping to be home soon. They were going to meet with the doctors and discuss the treatment plan for the balance of the week. I was still hopeful that I will be released for Christmas.

Chapter 21

RELEASED FROM THE HOSPITAL

THURSDAY, DECEMBER 14, 1978. I UNDERWENT ANOTHER SERIES of X-rays in the morning. Then, that same afternoon, the doctors informed me that I could call my parents to pick me up. I would be home for Christmas. I was given a strict list of instructions of all the things that I could not do. I had to wear the Philadelphia Collar twenty-four hours a day, only being allowed to take it off for a short shower. I was starting to feel better. The pressure on my neck and head seemed to have eased, and there was very little tingling in my hands and feet.

Finally, I could swallow without choking and I started, slowly, to gain back some weight. The doctors would not allow me to go back to school until after the holiday season. I was still extremely weak and had very little color, but in reality, I was feeling better.

Dr. Ebersold informed me that there is no way possible that I could play football again, but he left open the possibility of playing other sports… if the neck fusion healed correctly.

Sacred Heart Hospital had become a second home to me. I could not wait to get back home and sleep in my own bed—without a body cast. On the ride back to Durand, my parents were concerned with the amount of school I'd missed and apparently the discussion of repeating my junior year of high school had come up again.

I told my parents that I would do make-up school work through the holiday in attempt to get caught up. Joe Plumer and other classmates had collected homework assignments for me and brought my school books to my house. I turned in some make-up work before Christmas and took some make-up tests over the holiday. The teaching staff was excellent and supportive. I was eager to return to school and start the new year of 1979.

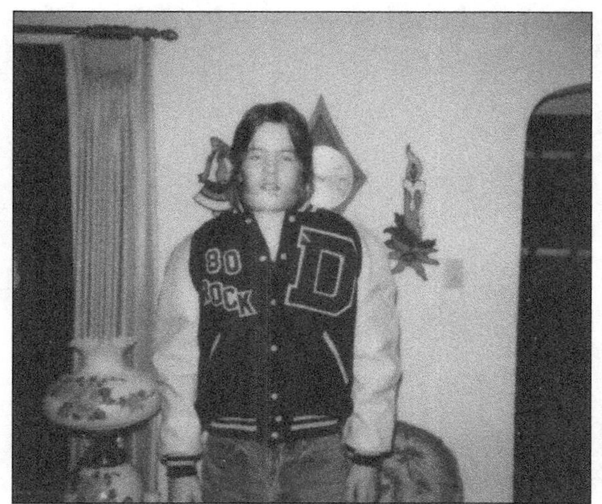

Returning home after second surgery in a cervical collar.

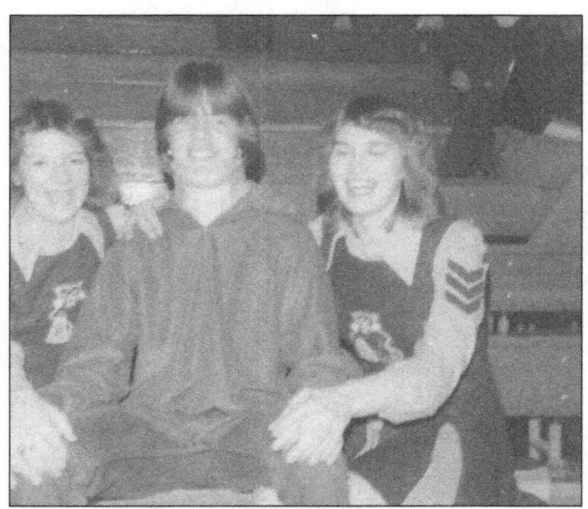

Two Durand cheerleaders bring a smile to my face.

Chapter 22

LAST BREATH

THE ONE REGRET I HAVE IS THAT I DID NOT WRITE THIS BOOK WHILE my father was still alive. He was with me as much as he could be throughout my injury and recovery. My dad was a WWII veteran and fought in several battles in the Marshall Islands. He was in the battle of Tarawa, Roi-Namur, and was also stationed on Guam and Saipan. Dad joined the service in 1943, at the age of seventeen, while still in high school. Growing up in the great depression of the 1930s, he had very few luxuries in life. Times were tough. His mother was an invalid. She was paralyzed at the time of my father's birth. He never once had seen his own mother walk. The only mother he'd ever known lived in a wheelchair.

Worse yet, his father, Romeo, left the family when he was about three years old, so he never really knew his Dad. Romeo only came to visit a few times and my Dad had very little memory of him, just a few old photos. Imagine as a young child, you have no father and your mother is paralyzed and in a wheelchair. This is the description of *tough*.

Sid Lunderville worked many hours, some people called him a workaholic. In the 1950s, he was deputized as a sheriff. He worked primarily the weekends, when his services were needed most. His main job was to respond to trouble and bar fights. The other policemen loved my dad, because there was not a fight he could not handle. He used his fists and a *Billy Club* to get the job done; no guns allowed.

His work day would begin very early, when he would help my mom and my brother, Scott, clean the bar from the previous night. Then he would head to his full-time job at Safeway, making powdered milk at the local factory. This was typically an eight-hour shift, or longer. After his full time job, he would come home, grab a sandwich, and he was back out the door, painting houses until dark. All the boys in our family learned how to paint, to earn money for college.

I did not get to see my dad as much as I wanted when I was young, but I got to spend more time with him when he finally retired. Most of that time was spent at his cottage on Big Round Lake.

His work ethic rubbed off on me, Dad really provided for a large family with a blue-collar job. Our family never went hungry. We didn't have a lot, but we seemed to have as much as others did, so we never complained or noticed that we lacked for anything. We were just a typical family of that era.

I always had the utmost respect for my Dad.

My father passed away June 19, 2015 at our family's cottage. It's a place he'd built with the help of his sons: Scott, Jeff, and Ross. His brother in law, Rudy Buchholtz, and his neighbor, Clarence Weissinger were also there swinging a hammer.

Dad *took his last breath as my mother and I held him.* His time had come… his heart was weak and failing, and he was about to turn ninety years old. His wish was to pass at the cabin he'd built.

His wish had come true.

Some of his ashes were spread on Big Round Lake, in Wisconsin. As close relatives, children, grandchildren, and great-grandchildren gathered on pontoons and motor boats to bid him farewell. His granddaughter, Alexis Weisser, recited the perfect poem for the occasion. It was so fitting that Donna, Sid's wife, still recites it from memory every day.

To Those Whom I Love & Those Who Love Me

When I am gone, release me, let me go.
I have so many things to see and do,
You mustn't tie yourself to me with too many tears,
But be thankful we had so many good years.

I gave you my love, and you can only guess
How much you've given me in happiness.
I thank you for the love that you have shown,
But now it is time I traveled on alone.

So, grieve for me a while, if grieve you must,
Then let your grief be comforted by trust.
It is only for a while that we must part,
So treasure the memories within your heart.

I won't be far away for life goes on.
And if you need me, call and I will come.

Though you can't see or touch me, I will be near.
And if you listen with your heart, you'll hear,
All my love around you soft and clear.

And then, when you come this way alone,
I'll greet you with a smile and a "Welcome Home."

Author: Anonymous

Following the beautiful verses, flowers from the funeral had been lobbed off and handed out, to mostly the great-grandchildren present. The powdery ashes dispersed quickly as the wind swept them through the air and over the rippling water around us. That was the cue for the great-grandchildren to drop their flowers onto the water's surface. White daisies, chrysanthemums, and carnations floated gently on the water. Lingering around, unlike the ashes, they gave us all a moment to reflect on the events and offer our final goodbyes to a wonderful brother-in-law, father, and father-in-law, granddad, and great-granddad.

Until we meet again Dad; the cottage is in good hands and being taken care of just like I promised.

CONCLUSION

I AM EXTREMELY LUCKY TO BE WALKING TODAY. I THANK THE LORD and Doctor Mike Ebersold for that. If it were not for both, I would not be here today. Doctor Ebersold is the one who recognized that my neck was, in fact, broke. He became one of the top neurosurgeons at the Mayo Clinic in Rochester, Minnesota. Although the first attempt with the halo traction failed, the neck fusion was successful.

A former actor and accomplished horseman, Christopher Reeves, best known for his movie role as "Superman," broke his top two cervical vertebrae. He was not so lucky and was permanently paralyzed. I remember reading the articles. "As actor Christopher Reeves remained paralyzed and unable to breathe on his own five days after breaking his neck in an equestrian accident, experts in spinal cord injuries said Thursday that the circumstances—breaks high in the spinal column—indicate a potentially devastating injury, among the worst imaginable." *June 2, 1995 Los Angeles Times by Marlene Cimons*

I read and realized just how lucky I was to have broken C1 and C2 and escaped without severing my spinal cord. Only one more hit or one more tackle and I could have been in a wheelchair for the rest of my life. If it were not for the persistence of my teammates forcing me to leave the huddle, I may have kept playing that night. I have always told Marty Weiss, our senior linebacker on the team, that he may have saved my life. I will never forget his words, "Get him the hell out of here." I can visualize that moment in my mind yet today.

In 1989, I read an article about Dr. Mike Ebersold removing a tumor on the brain of President Ronald Reagan. Looking back, I was blessed with a very good doctor. My life could have been totally different and filled with numerous and much worse challenges. Sure, I have physical limitations, but for the most part have led a normal life. I attempted to play some basketball and baseball my senior year in high school with limited success. I had to play basketball with a cervical collar; it limited my range of motion making it difficult to shoot the ball. I did not have all my balance back and there was still some numbness in my hands and feet. I was not the athlete I once was.

I am blessed to have a lovely and supportive wife Karla (Fedie) Lunderville. We married in 1984 in Lima, a small rural community near Durand. She continually reminded me to document and write down all the things that happened to me from my accident, so I did. I have scribbled notes, an old cassette tape I had recorded, and some of the notes I kept when I was in the hospital. Her persistence encouraged me to write this book. Forty years later and I can still recall almost every event that happened.

After several moves, my wife and I settled in Green Bay, Wisconsin, where we raised two beautiful daughters: Alexis Weisser and Aubrey Lunderville. I am extremely proud of both of them and their accomplishments. I cannot imagine my life without my family. I remember telling my story for the first time to both of them; they were very young. They were both very startled when I told them the details. They became scared when I showed them the scars on the back of my neck, and my hip where they took bone grafts.

The truth be told, during my accident and all the way through recovery, I always tried to put on a smile. Under my smile there was pain, constant pain, but I always tried to stay positive. I had pain before I broke my neck, and pain from the surgeries and the recovery process. I still have very limited neck motion today, but I have made the best of it.

There was no *concussion protocol* back in 1978. When you were knocked out or could not think straight, "You had your bell rung." I am glad that things have changed. I have no regrets and do not fault any of my coaches or doctors. It happened. The coaches of that time were not educated on concussions or any sort of protocol. I also ignored some warning signs—again, I was unsure of what was happening, I was only sixteen-years old and had never seen anyone experience this type of injury. I put on a tough exterior for my family and myself through the grueling treatment and healing process and then unknown outcome.

I remember people asking me if my parents were going to file a lawsuit against the local hospital and the doctors in my hometown of Durand. The answer was a simple "No." My parents did not believe a lawsuit was the right thing to do. My father felt there were mistakes made, but none of them intentional. I supported my parents' decision. We did end up meeting with an attorney and he indicated that we had a legitimate lawsuit, but again my parents wanted nothing to do with it.

The high school athletes of today will probably not suffer the way I did. I had a couple of major concussions and should have been treated for them. My spinal cord had swollen to the point where I could not swallow. This was a scary sensation. Today there are doctors or certified trainers at most high school games; they are schooled in recognizing brain and neck trauma. There is *concussion protocol*.

I think as others read this book, they too, may know someone that went through what I did because, without precautions and protocols in place, these injuries occurred and went untreated.

Although my dream of playing college sports was over, there was still a life ahead of me.

I laid for over three days in the hospital, being treated for a sprained neck, only to find out it was actually fractured vertebrae. Then, another five days before surgery was scheduled. I believe that I played in four games with the injury and never knew it. *Really lucky...that's what I was*. One more hit, one more tackle, and I could have been permanently paralyzed and in a wheelchair.

To all the young athletes involved in sports, if you feel you are hurt or something is wrong in your body, do not be afraid to tell someone. When you notice something is hurting, get it checked, it is not worth the risk to further damage your body. Tell your team trainer or go see a doctor.

I have been a successful sales manager for over thirty-five years. Forty-one years have passed since my neck injury and concussions. I am now feeling some side effects, but I have always told myself this; "Somebody else has it worse than me."

Move forward and keep the Faith. God Bless.

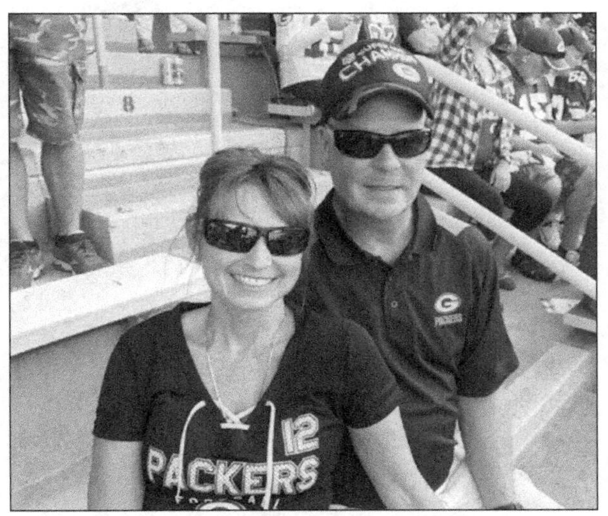

Brock and his wife Karla (2018)

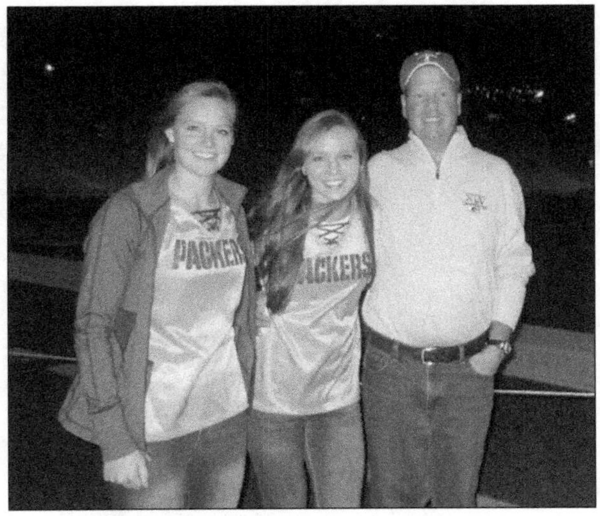

Brock and his daughters Alexis (L), and Aubrey (R) on Lambeau Field the night before a Green Bay Packer Game. (2016)

CPSIA information can be obtained
at www.ICGtesting.com
Printed in the USA
LVHW080152241019
635199LV00014B/127/P